THE POSITIVE PORTIONS

FOOD & FITNESS JOURNAL

Shannon Hammer

Fairview Press
Minneapolis

Published by Fairview Press, 2450 Riverside Avenue, Minneapolis, Minnesota 55454. Fairview Press is a division of Fairview Health Services, a community-focused health system, affiliated with the University of Minnesota, providing a complete range of services, from the prevention of illness and injury to care for the most complex medical conditions. For a free current catalog of Fairview Press titles, please call toll-free 1-800-544-8207. Or visit our Web site at www.fairviewpress.org.

Library of Congress Cataloging-in-Publication Data
Hammer, Shannon, 1969–
    The positive portions food and fitness journal / by Shannon Hammer.
        p. cm.
    ISBN 978-1-57749-228-3
    1. Weight loss. 2. Overweight persons—Diaries. I. Title.
    RM222.2.H22485 2010
    613.2'5—dc22
                                    2009029546

Printed in Canada
First Printing: January 2010
14   13   12   11   10   7   6   5   4   3   2   1

Cover design by Laurie Ingram
Interior design by Ryan Scheife, Mayfly Design (www.mayflydesign.net)

Medical Disclaimer:
This publication is designed to provide accurate and authoritative information in regard to the subject matter covered. It is sold with the understanding that neither the author nor the publisher is engaged in the provision or practice of medical, nursing, or professional healthcare advice or services in any jurisdiction. If medical advice or other professional assistance is required, the services of a qualified and competent professional should be sought. Neither Fairview Press nor the author is responsible or liable, directly or indirectly, for any form of damages whatsoever resulting from the use (or misuse) of information contained in or implied by these documents.

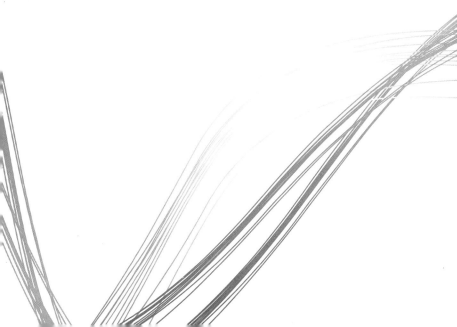

This book is dedicated to my mother, Eileen, the most generous person I have ever known; my husband, Mark, the person I want to be when I grow up; and all who seek wellness, one meal at a time.

*T*he *Positive Portions Food and Fitness Journal* is a little book with a big impact.

This six-month journal can help you achieve your health goals, whether you want to lose weight, increase your fitness, or improve your overall well-being. Combining the wisdom of a daily reflection book with the benefits of a food diary, this journal creates a custom experience unique to you—its pages invite you to document your food and activity levels, contemplate sage quotations, and engage in introspective exercises designed to keep you focused and motivated.

Research reported in the *American Journal of Preventive Medicine* (August 2008) found that people doubled their weight loss when they used a food journal. My own experience attests to the power of recording what you eat. After a lifetime of yo-yo dieting, I lost over 100 pounds and have kept it off by adopting a long-term, holistic approach to wellness that included writing down everything I ate.

Keeping a food journal was instrumental to my success—it provided me with the awareness and accountability I needed to take responsibility for my well-being. I was able to see exactly what, when, and how much I was eating, which helped me take positive action, such as planning meals in advance, eliminating trigger foods, and choosing healthy portions.

Taking care of my physical needs gave me insight into my emotional ones. I learned to identify when I was reaching for food not out of physical hunger but because of stress, fatigue, or emotions. I learned to curb impulsive eating and process my feelings in ways that didn't involve food, such as exercising, resting, and connecting with friends.

Even though I've been maintaining a healthy weight for several years now, I still keep a daily food journal as part of my lifelong commitment to wellness. I know that if keeping a food journal helped me achieve my goals, it can help you achieve yours.

I encourage you to dive into your journal, take charge of your health, and become your best self.

Warmly,

Shannon Hammer

Please visit www.PositivePortions.com.

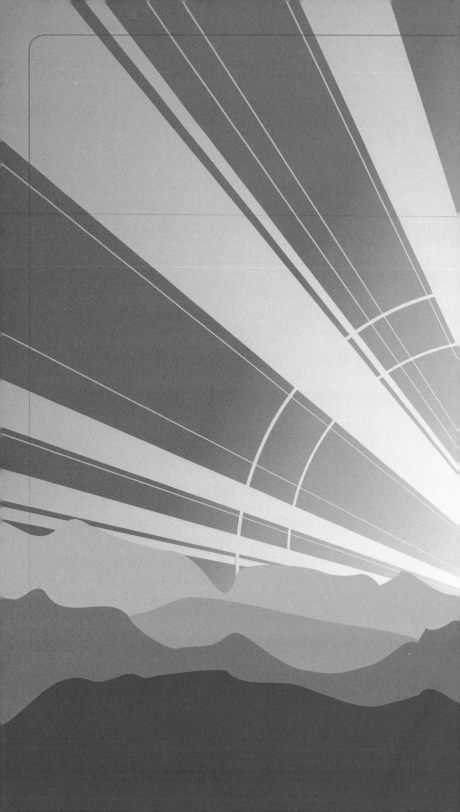

Month 1

Get Started

> "Today I start a diary; it is against my usual habits, but out of a clearly felt need."
>
> — Robert Musil

*O*ur daily fitness journals are powerful and important tools in helping us achieve wellness and reach our goals. When we diligently document our food and exercise, we can see exactly what, when, and how much we're eating and moving our bodies. We then have the information we need to track patterns, identify our vulnerable times, and discover what does and doesn't agree with our bodies.

To get the most out of our journals, it's important that we commit to 100 percent accountability. A good rule of thumb is this: If it has calories (or uses calories), it counts. From condiments to sauces to what we put in our coffee, it all needs to be written down. If we run a mile or spend fifteen minutes gardening, we need to write it down. The more thorough we are, the more we help ourselves succeed, and the healthier and happier we'll be.

Today, be accountable to yourself.

Daily Nutritional Information

Time	Amt.	Cal.	Fat gms	Protein gms	Carbs gms	Fiber gms
MORNING						
AFTERNOON						
EVENING						
TOTALS						

MY DAILY ACTIVITY

> *"Trying to improve something when you don't have a means of measurement and performance standards is like setting out on a cross-country trip in a car without a fuel gauge."*
>
> —◦ MIKEL HARRY

Sometimes we avoid looking in the mirror or stepping on a scale because we don't like how we look and we don't want to see the numbers. If we're going to become more fit, we need to know not only where we want to end up but also where we're starting from.

As painful as it may be, it's important to take an accurate assessment of what our physical state is, right here, right now. This means breaking out the measuring tape and stepping on the scale. Rather than feel embarrassed or shamed, we can view our numbers as starting points on a lifelong journey to health. We don't have to share the numbers with anyone; we just need to have them to track and celebrate our progress.

Today, weigh and measure yourself.

Daily Nutritional Information

Time	Amt.	Cal.	Fat gms	Protein gms	Carbs gms	Fiber gms
MORNING						
AFTERNOON						
EVENING						
TOTALS						

My Daily Activity

> "A vision is not just a picture of what could be; it is an appeal to our better selves, a call to become something more."
>
> —◐ ROSABETH MOSS KANTER

Creating a vision of wellness is more than declaring what number the scale should show, or how many repetitions (reps) we can do at the gym. What does wellness mean to us? How do we want to incorporate wellness in our daily routines on an ongoing basis? What do we think it will mean for our lives if we become fitter and healthier?

We need to have a vision that allows for real change.

Today, write down five wellness goals. What would you like to accomplish?

Daily Nutritional Information

Time	Amt.	Cal.	Fat gms	Protein gms	Carbs gms	Fiber gms
MORNING						
AFTERNOON						
EVENING						
TOTALS						

My Daily Activity

_____

_____

_____

_____

_____

_____

_____

_____

_____

"Blessed are those who hunger and thirst, for they are sticking to their diets."

—Anonymous

e just started a new food plan and we're starving. Is it all in our heads? Actually, no. Here's the bad news: At the onset of a new food plan, our body produces more of the hunger hormone ghrelin, which tells the brain when it's time to eat. Here's the good news: If we hang in there, our bodies will adjust and this initial hunger will wear off.

Although we don't want to set ourselves up for a binge by becoming too hungry, we also don't want to halt our progress by giving in to the grumbling of our stomachs too easily. The way to survive is to remind ourselves that hunger is temporary and that this, too, shall pass.

Today, keep your eyes on long-term results rather than any short-term discomfort.

Daily Nutritional Information

Time	Amt.	Cal.	Fat gms	Protein gms	Carbs gms	Fiber gms
MORNING						
AFTERNOON						
EVENING						
TOTALS						

MY DAILY ACTIVITY

_____

_____

_____

_____

_____

_____

_____

_____

_____

"If you'll not settle for anything less than your best, you will be amazed at what you can accomplish in your lives."

—VINCE LOMBARDI

Wellness isn't about settling for less; it's about setting goals for what we really want and taking our best action to achieve them. Our goals are as diverse as we are. Some of us want to run marathons, others want to get back into clothes we haven't been able to wear for years, and still others dream of walking up flights of stairs without being winded. Whatever our personal goals, they are worthy of our best efforts.

Today, don't settle for anything less than your best to get what you really want.

Daily Nutritional Information

Time	Amt.	Cal.	Fat gms	Protein gms	Carbs gms	Fiber gms
MORNING						
AFTERNOON						
EVENING						
TOTALS						

My Daily Activity

_____

_____

_____

_____

_____

_____

_____

_____

_____

> *"Nothing would be more tiresome than eating and drinking if God had not made them a pleasure as well as a necessity."*
>
> —VOLTAIRE

*a*dopting a healthy lifestyle doesn't mean we can't still enjoy eating; a key component to successful healthy living is to eat food that nourishes both our bodies and our palates.

If we dislike the food we're eating, then we're eating the wrong food. The world is filled with enough resources—grocery and health food stores, restaurants and farmers' markets—to accommodate our personal preferences while still supporting our wellness goals. When we love what we eat, we will be more likely to stick to our programs . . . joyfully.

Today, eat food you love.

Daily Nutritional Information

Time	Amt.	Cal.	Fat gms	Protein gms	Carbs gms	Fiber gms
MORNING						
AFTERNOON						
EVENING						
TOTALS						

MY DAILY ACTIVITY

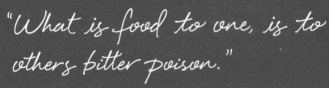

"What is food to one, is to others bitter poison."

—⌒ LUCRETIUS

Wouldn't it be nice if we only had healthy, nourishing food in our homes? Many of us don't have that option because we live with people who eat food that's fine for them but not good for us. How can we share our space and still eat only the food we know is good for us?

The trick is to remind ourselves that the unhealthy food in our homes isn't ours. Just as the people we live with have items like clothing and shoes that don't belong to us, they also have food that doesn't belong to us. When we open the refrigerator and see temptation, repeating supportive statements such as "That's not my food" can help us stay focused on the healthy food that is ours.

Today, share your space, not your food.

Daily Nutritional Information

Time	Amt.	Cal.	Fat gms	Protein gms	Carbs gms	Fiber gms
MORNING						
AFTERNOON						
EVENING						
TOTALS						

MY DAILY ACTIVITY

_____

_____

_____

_____

_____

_____

_____

_____

_____

_____

"The name of the game is taking care of yourself, because you're going to live long enough to wish you had."

—᧕ GRACE MIRABELLA

or many of us, the issue isn't taking care of our weight or health; it's taking care of ourselves. We spend so much time taking care of others that we forget about ourselves. If we want to attain and maintain wellness, we will have to learn how to put ourselves at the top of the priority list.

We may mistake self-care for selfishness. Healthy self-care simply means we place as much value on ourselves as we do on other people. We recognize that we deserve the same care and attention as everybody else. We acknowledge our own worth. It's up to us to become our own best advocate.

Today, put yourself on your priority list.

Daily Nutritional Information

Time	Amt.	Cal.	Fat gms	Protein gms	Carbs gms	Fiber gms
MORNING						
AFTERNOON						
EVENING						
TOTALS						

My Daily Activity

_____

_____

_____

_____

_____

_____

_____

_____

_____

"The large print giveth and the small print taketh away."

—ᏆᎾᎷ Waits

When was the last time we read the small print on packaged foods? Food labels, those little sections of information on every box, package, or bag, contain more information than just calories and fat grams—they also tell us whether the foods that are advertised in the large print as "healthy" really are.

The true test of a product's value lies in the small print under "ingredients." This is where we can see what's *really* in the food, such as hidden sugars, preservatives, and dyes. A good rule of thumb to determine whether a food supports our wellness goals is to look past the large print and trust the small print instead.

Today, read your labels.

Daily Nutritional Information

Time	Amt.	Cal.	Fat gms	Protein gms	Carbs gms	Fiber gms
MORNING						
AFTERNOON						
EVENING						
TOTALS						

MY DAILY ACTIVITY

"The most remarkable thing about my mother is that for thirty years she served the family nothing but leftovers. The original meal has never been found."

—◦ CALVIN TRILLIN

W e may be the only ones in our households trying to live a healthier life, but that doesn't mean we have to go it alone. Why not make wellness a family affair? We can include our loved ones by incorporating healthy practices into our daily activities.

Shopping for healthy food can be enjoyable if we ask our loved ones to join us and select fresh produce and other items they like. We can share the ups and downs of our days while we work together to prepare a good meal. Walks in the park, trips to the baseball diamond, or afternoon bike rides are great opportunities to have quality time while getting in exercise we need. With a little creativity, sharing our wellness can be practical, simple, and fun.

Today, find ways to share your wellness with loved ones.

Daily Nutritional Information

Time	Amt.	Cal.	Fat gms	Protein gms	Carbs gms	Fiber gms
MORNING						
AFTERNOON						
EVENING						
TOTALS						

My Daily Activity

_____

_____

_____

_____

_____

_____

_____

_____

_____

> *"You may have to fight a battle more than once to win it."*
>
> — MARGARET THATCHER

Conquering unhealthy habits is a battle we may need to fight more than once in order to win. Old habits die hard; feelings come up, and setbacks happen. If we want to triumph over bad habits like surrendering to a sneak attack of nighttime eating or spending our free time exercising only the remote control, we need to break out the big guns: patience and persistence.

We win the war when we patiently accept that lifelong patterns don't change overnight and persistently refuse to surrender. Every setback allows us to examine our battle scars, form new plans of attack, and get back on the battlefield. If we keep marching forward, we will ultimately be victorious.

Today, fight the good fight.

Daily Nutritional Information

Time	Amt.	Cal.	Fat gms	Protein gms	Carbs gms	Fiber gms
MORNING						
AFTERNOON						
EVENING						
TOTALS						

MY DAILY ACTIVITY

_____

_____

_____

_____

_____

_____

_____

_____

_____

> *"Technology does not drive change—it enables change."*
>
> —⌘ ANONYMOUS

*L*iving in the digital age has its advantages. Not only can we merge companies with the click of a mouse and watch a movie in the car, we also can use twenty-first-century technology to get some good old-fashioned exercise.

Technology gives us tools to work out wherever we are. We can download videos onto our laptops and MP3 players and exercise in hotel rooms. We can pop exercise videos into our DVD players and get fit in the living room. We can put on headphones and hit the sidewalk, park, or hiking trail. A little technology, combined with a lot of motivation, can help us stay fit and healthy no matter where the information highway takes us.

Today, use technology to help meet your goals.

Daily Nutritional Information

Time	Amt.	Cal.	Fat gms	Protein gms	Carbs gms	Fiber gms
MORNING						
AFTERNOON						
EVENING						
TOTALS						

MY DAILY ACTIVITY

_____

_____

_____

_____

_____

_____

_____

_____

_____

_____

> *"Coming together, sharing together, working together, succeeding together."*
>
> —ᴄⱾ Aɴᴏɴʏᴍᴏᴜs

We increase our chances of success when we connect to a wellness community—a group of others working toward the same goal. Not only do we benefit from forming supportive relationships with fellow seekers, we also benefit from the experience, strength, and hope of people who have gained better health and wellness.

With a little effort, we can easily tap into wellness communities, both in person and online. If we have a specific interest, such as hiking or walking, we can look into joining groups that meet regularly. We may find the support we need in chat rooms, blogs, or social networking sites. Or we may enjoy the camaraderie of a gym or yoga studio. How we connect is less important than that we are connecting.

Today, tap into a wellness community.

Daily Nutritional Information

Time	Amt.	Cal.	Fat gms	Protein gms	Carbs gms	Fiber gms
MORNING						
AFTERNOON						
EVENING						
TOTALS						

MY DAILY ACTIVITY

"The ability to discipline yourself to delay gratification in the short term in order to enjoy greater rewards in the long term is the indispensable prerequisite for success."

—◇ BRIAN TRACY

*a*t times sticking to our wellness goals will require us to say no to things that make us feel good now but terrible later. At these times, we need to stay strong by reminding ourselves that we're not really giving anything up—we're making room for something better.

We may have to say no to unhealthy favorite foods and yes to foods that nourish us but aren't as exciting. In reality, we're trading in foods that promote disease for ones that encourage healing. We may have to give up our couch-potato lifestyle and start exercising. In reality, we're trading in weak muscles and stiffness for strength and stamina. Success can be ours when we keep our eye on the big picture—and practice a little delayed gratification.

Today, stay focused on long-term rewards.

Daily Nutritional Information

Time	Amt.	Cal.	Fat gms	Protein gms	Carbs gms	Fiber gms
MORNING						
AFTERNOON						
EVENING						
TOTALS						

MY DAILY ACTIVITY

_____
_____
_____
_____
_____
_____
_____
_____
_____

> *"Some people go to priests; others to poetry; I to my friends."*
>
> —VIRGINIA WOOLF

*f*or many of us, food has been our best friend. Always available, easy to obtain, and inexpensive, food may have served as a steady Saturday night date, a comforting friend in a crisis, or a couch-side, TV-watching companion. Once we're living a healthier lifestyle, we need to find friendship in people, not packages. It's time to socialize.

Having a rich social life is part of a balanced life, whether our idea of socializing is a big party or a great one-on-one conversation. Friendships help banish loneliness and foster feelings of security, which strengthens our ability to stay on track with wellness and protect us against the effects of stress. We soon realize that the companionship we get from others nourishes us in ways food never could.

Today, reach out to a friend.

Daily Nutritional Information

Time	Amt.	Cal.	Fat gms	Protein gms	Carbs gms	Fiber gms
MORNING						
AFTERNOON						
EVENING						
TOTALS						

My Daily Activity

"Sour, sweet, bitter, pungent, all must be tasted."

—◦ CHINESE PROVERB

When we stick to a routine, we can get stuck in a rut. This is true in life, and it's true with our meals and our exercise. If we eat the same things over and over or run exactly the same path every day, we risk becoming bored and unmotivated. The key to keeping our interest in healthy eating is to eat a variety of delicious food. The key to getting our bodies stronger is doing different kinds of exercise.

Varying our menus gives us an opportunity to include new and different foods we might not have otherwise considered. Perhaps we'll incorporate juice, raw food, soup, or cuisine from exotic cultures. Maybe we'll discover a new twist on an old favorite. Varying our fitness routine gives us a chance to exercise different muscles and to discover new activities we enjoy.

Today, expand your options for diet and exercise.

Daily Nutritional Information

Time	Amt.	Cal.	Fat gms	Protein gms	Carbs gms	Fiber gms
MORNING						
AFTERNOON						
EVENING						
TOTALS						

My Daily Activity

_____

_____

_____

_____

_____

_____

_____

_____

_____

_____

> *"Repetition of the same thought or physical action develops into a habit which, repeated frequently enough, becomes an automatic reflex."*
>
> —Dr. Norman Vincent Peale

Habits don't just happen; we establish them through repetition. This means we can deliberately create the habits we want until they become automatic.

Just as we brush our teeth each day, almost without thinking about it, we can ingrain healthy habits with consistent, positive action. At first, we may have to push ourselves a bit, especially when we don't feel like it. We know we need to get fit, so we exercise whether or not we want to right now. We know we need to manage stress, so we meditate. Soon our new healthier habits become automatic reflexes; we just do them, no matter what.

Today, tap into the power of repetition.

Daily Nutritional Information

Time	Amt.	Cal.	Fat gms	Protein gms	Carbs gms	Fiber gms
MORNING						
AFTERNOON						
EVENING						
TOTALS						

MY DAILY ACTIVITY

"I just hate health food."

—JULIA CHILD

iguring out what to eat when we're trying to be healthy can be daunting, especially if we think of health food as being tasteless and boring. Fortunately, health-conscious people have been eating well for years and have perfected the art of creating healthy yet tasty meals. Why not tap into their experience and find recipes that fit both our programs and our preferences?

Resources are everywhere. The Internet connects us to Web sites, blogs, and online communities that offer information on everything from how to chop vegetables and prepare proteins to creating guilt-free desserts and healthy comfort foods. Bookstores are filled with specialty cookbooks. We can ask the healthy people we know to share some of their tried-and-true recipes. Meals we love that heal our bodies can be ours with a little effort.

Today, make healthy food delicious.

Daily Nutritional Information

Time	Amt.	Cal.	Fat gms	Protein gms	Carbs gms	Fiber gms
MORNING						
AFTERNOON						
EVENING						
TOTALS						

MY DAILY ACTIVITY

_____

_____

_____

_____

_____

_____

_____

_____

_____

> *"A quilt will warm your body and comfort your soul."*
>
> —Anonymous

We all have our favorite comfort foods, those foods we turn to when we're unhappy, stressed out, or missing home. But, when we think about it, are comfort foods really comforting? How comfortable do we end up feeling—emotionally or physically—when we overeat on heavy, starchy, or sugary foods? In the long run, comfort foods can make us feel very uncomfortable.

When we need comfort, we can find it in things other than food. We can listen to favorite old songs, take a fragrant bath or shower, walk until we're nicely exhausted, talk to a friend, take a nap under a warm quilt. Finding healthy avenues to feel better will soothe us now, comfortably.

Today, find ways to comfort yourself that don't involve food.

Daily Nutritional Information

Time	Amt.	Cal.	Fat gms	Protein gms	Carbs gms	Fiber gms
MORNING						
AFTERNOON						
EVENING						
TOTALS						

MY DAILY ACTIVITY

> *"No matter who you are,*
> *no matter what you do, you*
> *absolutely, positively do have*
> *the power to change."*
>
> —BILL PHILLIPS

No matter what our histories, we can change. If we've always had a troubled relationship with food, we don't have to keep that up. If we've always been couch potatoes, we can become active.

If we've learned unhealthy eating habits, we can learn new ones. If we haven't exercised in years, we can start. As long as there is breath in our bodies, there is hope.

Today, yes you can.

Daily Nutritional Information

Time	Amt.	Cal.	Fat gms	Protein gms	Carbs gms	Fiber gms
MORNING						
AFTERNOON						
EVENING						
TOTALS						

MY DAILY ACTIVITY

> "I refuse to become part of this perfect-body syndrome. I like my body. It looks good onscreen, and it's not because it's perfect. I accept it and wear it like a good dress."
>
> —*Salma Hayek*

There's no such thing as a perfect body. We do ourselves a great disservice when we unfairly compare ourselves to models and celebrities who have been done-up, made-up, and blown-dry. An important part of our journey to good health is to let go of the unrealistic quest for perfection and accept our bodies with all of their curves, bumps, and freckles.

The first step to self-acceptance is to take care of ourselves. We'll feel better and look our best, whatever that is. Then we can more easily appreciate and love our bodies in all their real-life glory.

Today, accept your body as it is.

Daily Nutritional Information

Time	Amt.	Cal.	Fat gms	Protein gms	Carbs gms	Fiber gms
MORNING						
AFTERNOON						
EVENING						
TOTALS						

MY DAILY ACTIVITY

_____

_____

_____

_____

_____

_____

_____

_____

_____

"My drug of choice is food."

—⟡ OPRAH WINFREY

Many of us use food as the alcoholic uses alcohol—to cope, comfort, console. Unlike the alcoholic, however, we can't just stop eating. How can we best control our use of something we have to consume to live?

In order not to abuse food, we need to be fully conscious of every bite. This is why keeping a food journal, establishing a wellness community, and developing our emotional and spiritual lives is so important—we need these tools to help us stay present, focused, and balanced.

Today, use your tools.

Daily Nutritional Information

Time	Amt.	Cal.	Fat gms	Protein gms	Carbs gms	Fiber gms
MORNING						
AFTERNOON						
EVENING						
TOTALS						

My Daily Activity

_____

_____

_____

_____

_____

_____

_____

_____

_____

> *"Fitness—if it came in a bottle, everybody would have a great body."*
>
> —CHER

Wouldn't it be great to be fit without exercising or watching what we eat? Sometimes it seems as if others can do just that, and maybe, given the body type and metabolism they were born with, they can. But we know that we are going to have to work at it.

There's no shortcut to fitness, but the good news is that the things we do to become fit—eating healthy foods, getting plenty of sleep, exercising regularly, drinking lots of water—will do more than make our bodies look better. Being fit physically helps us be fit mentally and emotionally as well.

Today, do what you know you need to.

Daily Nutritional Information

Time	Amt.	Cal.	Fat gms	Protein gms	Carbs gms	Fiber gms
MORNING						
AFTERNOON						
EVENING						
TOTALS						

My Daily Activity

_____

_____

_____

_____

_____

_____

_____

_____

_____

> *"As a child, my family's menu consisted of two choices: take it or leave it."*
>
> —☙ BUDDY HACKETT

*E*arly in our lives, we form our beliefs about food based on what we are taught, the eating habits of those around us, and our early environments. As adults, we get to reexamine our early programming and decide for ourselves which beliefs serve us today and which ones don't.

Maybe we were taught that not finishing everything on our plates was wasteful. Now we can see that eating food our body doesn't need is also wasteful. Perhaps we had to eat everything served to us, whether we liked it or not. Now we can serve ourselves food we like in portions that are right for us. As adults, we have the power to take charge of our health and create new beliefs about food.

Today, identify and discard early beliefs about food that don't serve you anymore.

Daily Nutritional Information

Time	Amt.	Cal.	Fat gms	Protein gms	Carbs gms	Fiber gms
MORNING						
AFTERNOON						
EVENING						
TOTALS						

MY DAILY ACTIVITY

_____

_____

_____

_____

_____

_____

_____

_____

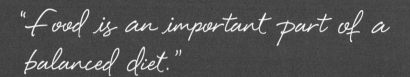

"Food is an important part of a balanced diet."

—ᥫ Fran Lebowitz

*H*ow many of us have been on diets that required we consume only powders, pills, or shakes? We paid good money to eat engineered food that not only didn't produce lasting results but also wreaked havoc with our social lives—how can we join our friends for dinner if we're not eating? One of the benefits of working toward holistic wellness is that we get to . . . eat. Food.

Instead of consuming food substitutes, we eat real, healthy, satisfying food. We can join our loved ones at restaurants, barbeques, and potlucks and be part of the group. We not only get to eat food we like, we also get the lasting results we want.

Today, eat and enjoy your food.

Daily Nutritional Information

Time	Amt.	Cal.	Fat gms	Protein gms	Carbs gms	Fiber gms
MORNING						
AFTERNOON						
EVENING						
TOTALS						

MY DAILY ACTIVITY

_____
_____
_____
_____
_____
_____
_____
_____
_____

"There is a charm about the forbidden that makes it unspeakably desirable."

—Ⓢ MARK TWAIN

*a*t times, going to a restaurant is a trip to temptation. From the appetizers to the desserts, delicious dishes entice us to forget about watching calories and fat. We can reduce temptation and increase our chances of eating healthfully if we proactively review the menu beforehand and preselect two meals—a first choice and a backup, just in case.

Not giving ourselves the option to choose a meal in the moment lessens the chances we'll make impulsive choices we'll regret later. When we come prepared with a plan, we don't even have to open the menu. We can concentrate on enjoying our companion's conversation instead of worrying about our meal.

Today, be proactive.

Daily Nutritional Information

Time	Amt.	Cal.	Fat gms	Protein gms	Carbs gms	Fiber gms
MORNING						
AFTERNOON						
EVENING						
TOTALS						

MY DAILY ACTIVITY

"The most successful people are those who are good at Plan B."

—⌒ JAMES YORKE

Life is in session—deadlines loom, the kids have soccer, and the boss just volunteered us for the next big project. When, exactly, are we supposed to exercise? When life disrupts our workout schedules, what we need is a Plan B.

Plan B is an alternative solution to getting exercise when life thwarts Plan A. Plan Bs usually consist of "if . . . then" statements and allow us to fit exercise into a disrupted schedule. *If I can't make it to the gym after work, then I'll take a walk during my lunch break. If the laundry is piled up, then I'll do an exercise video at home while washing clothes.* Plan Bs let us to take control of our schedules when life interferes.

Today, have a Plan B.

Daily Nutritional Information

Time	Amt.	Cal.	Fat gms	Protein gms	Carbs gms	Fiber gms
MORNING						
AFTERNOON						
EVENING						
TOTALS						

MY DAILY ACTIVITY

> *"Food is, delightfully, an area of licensed sensuality, of physical delight which will, with luck and enduring taste buds, last our life long."*
>
> —ꙮ ANTONIA TILL

*W*hat is more stimulating to the appetite than the five senses? The smell of freshly baked goods, the sight of the dessert tray, or the sizzling sound of food on a grill can flip a switch in our brains and make us want to eat—whether we're truly hungry or not.

Eating is meant to be a full-sensory experience, but our senses can trigger impulses to eat food our bodies don't need. One trick to combat this is to limit our exposure to food when it's not time for a meal. At parties, we can mingle with people rather than lingering near the food table. We can steer clear of the bakery section in grocery stores. Then, when it is time to eat, we can enjoy the sight, smell, taste, touch, and sound of every healthy bite.

Today, pay attention to your senses at mealtime.

Daily Nutritional Information

Time	Amt.	Cal.	Fat gms	Protein gms	Carbs gms	Fiber gms
MORNING						
AFTERNOON						
EVENING						
TOTALS						

MY DAILY ACTIVITY

"An hour of basketball feels like fifteen minutes. An hour on a treadmill feels like a weekend in traffic school."

—David Walters

*W*ho says exercise has to happen in a gym? If we're looking for a way to get fit that doesn't involve weights, locker rooms, or monthly fees, team sports may be a perfect solution.

Along with providing fun social ways to get fresh air, activity, and friendship, team sports can be a good way to improve our overall mental health. We tap into the team's energy to give us the strength and determination to safely push ourselves past our limits and achieve new goals. Better yet, we may be having so much fun that we forget we're exercising.

Today, consider participating in a team sport.

Daily Nutritional Information

Time	Amt.	Cal.	Fat gms	Protein gms	Carbs gms	Fiber gms
MORNING						
AFTERNOON						
EVENING						
TOTALS						

MY DAILY ACTIVITY

"Setting an example is not the main means of influencing another, it is the only means."

—ALBERT EINSTEIN

After embarking on a journey of wellness, we may feel so good emotionally and physically that we want everyone to do what we're doing. They would just feel so much better, we think, if they would eat right and exercise. We're right: Most people do feel better when they take care of ourselves. It's not our job, however, to monitor other people's behavior. The only behavior we can monitor is our own.

The best way to inspire people to take care of themselves is to be an example. When we take care of ourselves, our own health, happiness, and well-being will say more to those around us than any words we could use.

Today, let your health speak for itself.

Daily Nutritional Information

Time	Amt.	Cal.	Fat gms	Protein gms	Carbs gms	Fiber gms
MORNING						
AFTERNOON						
EVENING						
TOTALS						

My Daily Activity

_____

_____

_____

_____

_____

_____

_____

_____

_____

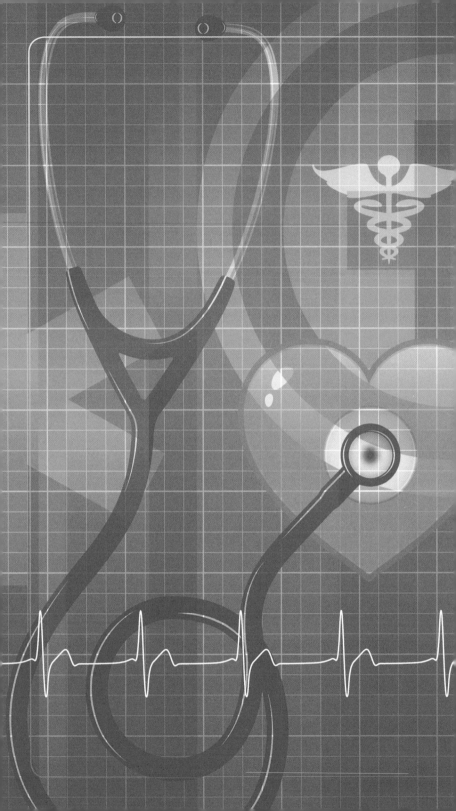

Month 2

Establish Healthy Habits

"Celebrate any progress. Don't wait to get perfect."

—ANN McGEE COOPER

C hanging lifestyles is quite a feat—growth and progress are unpredictable, nonlinear processes. Most of us dismiss incremental improvement as "not counting." If we lose two pounds instead of the five we wanted, the two pounds "don't count." If we walk twenty minutes instead of the sixty we intended, the twenty minutes "don't count."

This type of thinking simply won't do. Every bit of progress we make counts. We need to celebrate incremental success and believe that any improvement—no matter how small—is the beginning of a trend. This is how we make ourselves healthy, one small step at a time.

Today, remind yourself that every positive action counts.

Daily Nutritional Information

Time	Amt.	Cal.	Fat gms	Protein gms	Carbs gms	Fiber gms
MORNING						
AFTERNOON						
EVENING						
TOTALS						

My Daily Activity

_____

_____

_____

_____

_____

_____

_____

_____

_____

> *"Whenever I feel like exercise, I lie down until the feeling passes."*
>
> —⟊ ROBERT M. HUTCHINS

For some of us, the word "exercise" is synonymous with "torture." Fortunately, there is hope for the exercise averse. The trick is to tap into what we already love and find ways to use it to make our bodies move.

Music fans may want to join a dance class or buy a how-to dance video. Outdoorsy types can find scenic trails to hike or take to the streets on bicycles or roller skates. We can add exercise to activities we already love doing. If we love to garden, for example, we can stretch our upper bodies and practice leg-strengthening squats while pulling weeds. The key is to work with what we already enjoy.

Today, make exercise fun.

Daily Nutritional Information

Time	Amt.	Cal.	Fat gms	Protein gms	Carbs gms	Fiber gms
MORNING						
AFTERNOON						
EVENING						
TOTALS						

MY DAILY ACTIVITY

"You have to get right back on the horse that threw you."

—⟡ AMERICAN SAYING

Okay, we blew it: We gave in to that unhealthy food that was calling our name. Or maybe we got busy and didn't make it to our exercise class. Since we already blew it, we might as well just eat whatever we want, skip the gym, and start again tomorrow, right? That thinking is like a person getting a speeding ticket in the morning and then deciding to break all traffic laws for the rest of the day: It doesn't make sense in light of the damage that could occur.

The longer we wait to get back on track, the harder it will be. We owe it to ourselves to get back on the path to our goals right now, not tomorrow or next week.

Today, if you fall off your fitness plan, pick yourself up and start again.

Daily Nutritional Information

Time	Amt.	Cal.	Fat gms	Protein gms	Carbs gms	Fiber gms
MORNING						
AFTERNOON						
EVENING						
TOTALS						

MY DAILY ACTIVITY

"Learning is not attained by chance; it must be sought for with ardor and diligence."

—⌇ ABIGAIL ADAMS

Just as we need to feed our bodies a healthy diet of food, we also need to feed our minds a healthy diet of learning. Education doesn't occur only in a classroom, nor does it end after graduation. If we commit to being lifelong learners, the world becomes an ever-expanding classroom of continuous education.

We grow when we ardently and diligently seek new knowledge. Educational opportunities abound. We are always surrounded with countless new subjects to explore, new skills to acquire, and new challenges to meet.

Today, learn something new.

Daily Nutritional Information

Time	Amt.	Cal.	Fat gms	Protein gms	Carbs gms	Fiber gms
MORNING						
AFTERNOON						
EVENING						
TOTALS						

MY DAILY ACTIVITY

> "I watched the Indy 500, and I was thinking that if they left earlier they wouldn't have to go so fast."
>
> —<small>STEVEN WRIGHT</small>

*a*re we always rushing around? Sometimes we need to rush, such as when we need to catch a flight or have a tight deadline, but constant rushing has a negative impact on our physical, mental, and spiritual health.

The constant stream of adrenaline wears us down, making us prone to illness and fatigue and preventing us from fully relaxing. Rushing also robs us of our peace of mind and ability to stay in the present.

If we're to find balance, we need to keep our rushing to a minimum. This can mean scheduling fewer appointments, delegating tasks, and yes, even leaving work earlier.

Today, avoid the rush.

Daily Nutritional Information

Time	Amt.	Cal.	Fat gms	Protein gms	Carbs gms	Fiber gms
MORNING						
AFTERNOON						
EVENING						
TOTALS						

My Daily Activity

"It pays to plan ahead. It wasn't raining when Noah built the ark."

—Anonymous

The old adage is true: If we fail to plan, we plan to fail. Planning is especially important on those days when we we're facing a jam-packed or complicated schedule.

At the start of the day, we need to consider what's ahead and plan accordingly. If we know we have a long car trip ahead, we can pack lunch rather than rely on roadside fast-food restaurants. If we know we are going to be working late, we can bring nutritious snacks so that hunger doesn't drive us to the vending machines. If we know we'll miss our normal walk, we can pop an exercise DVD in first thing in the morning. When we take charge of our schedules, we take charge of our health.

Today, plan to succeed.

Daily Nutritional Information

Time	Amt.	Cal.	Fat gms	Protein gms	Carbs gms	Fiber gms
MORNING						
AFTERNOON						
EVENING						
TOTALS						

MY DAILY ACTIVITY

"All happiness depends on a leisurely breakfast."

—JOHN GUNTHER

Many of us treat eating as if it were a race against time. We inhale breakfast, nose-dive into lunch, and wolf down dinner. Slowing down brings awareness to our eating, which helps us learn when we're really hungry, when we're full, and what food feels good in our bodies.

Not rushing allows us to fully experience the flavor of our meals. We may be surprised to discover we feel full with less food, or perhaps we'll learn that we're not eating enough. We learn we like food less spicy or more. The point is to pause, pay attention, and be present.

Today, eat mindfully.

Daily Nutritional Information

Time	Amt.	Cal.	Fat gms	Protein gms	Carbs gms	Fiber gms
MORNING						
AFTERNOON						
EVENING						
TOTALS						

MY DAILY ACTIVITY

> "There is a spiritual hunger in the world today and it cannot be satisfied by better cars on longer credit terms."
>
> —⟳ADLAI E. STEVENSON

Our meal is done, our plate is empty, and we're still hungry—now what? If we've just eaten a healthy, satisfying meal, chances are our hunger isn't physical, it's emotional or spiritual. Now it's up to us to keep our forks down and feed ourselves in other ways.

First, we need to ask ourselves what we are really hungry for: love? attention? comfort? Once we've identified our true need, we can take positive action, such as journaling, talking to a friend, going for a walk . . . or even just sitting still with our feelings until they pass. Separating and identifying our different hungers allows us to give ourselves true nourishment, not unnecessary food.

Today, identify your real hunger.

Daily Nutritional Information

Time	Amt.	Cal.	Fat gms	Protein gms	Carbs gms	Fiber gms
MORNING						
AFTERNOON						
EVENING						
TOTALS						

My Daily Activity

_____

_____

_____

_____

_____

_____

_____

_____

_____

> *"We must make the choices that enable us to fulfill the deepest capacities of our real selves."*
>
> —⁂ THOMAS MERTON

Despite our best planning and careful preparation, we are going to encounter situations in which we aren't going to have a lot of healthy choices. Perhaps we're traveling, attending business events, or staying with friends. We don't have much control over the food presented to us or whether we can fit exercise into our schedule. In these cases, we simply need to make the best choices we can for the situation we're in.

We also have to be careful not to allow limited choices to be an excuse to disregard our healthy habits entirely. To offset impulsiveness, we can examine our food selections before we eat. Are we making the best possible choice we can? Can we modify a meal to make it healthier? Can we do an exercise routine in our room, or use a nearby health club for a short workout? If we're satisfied we're doing our best, we can do what we need to and then get to our healthy routines as soon as possible.

Today, make the best possible choices.

Daily Nutritional Information

Time	Amt.	Cal.	Fat gms	Protein gms	Carbs gms	Fiber gms
MORNING						
AFTERNOON						
EVENING						
TOTALS						

MY DAILY ACTIVITY

> "There are two reasons for drinking: one is, when you are thirsty, to cure it; the other, when you are not thirsty, to prevent it."
>
> —<small>⊳</small> THOMAS LOVE PEACOCK

Thirst often disguises itself as hunger. What may be a hankering for food is really a need for water. Keeping ourselves hydrated is not only good for our overall health, it also can help soothe the false cravings that tempt us to eat food we don't need.

There are ways to simply and easily stay hydrated. We can make it a habit to drink a bottle of water on the way to and from work. We can grab a glass when we refill our coffee cup. If plain water doesn't appeal to us, we can drink herbal teas or add fresh fruit juice. We may find it's easier to eat less by drinking more.

Today, stay hydrated.

Daily Nutritional Information

Time	Amt.	Cal.	Fat gms	Protein gms	Carbs gms	Fiber gms
MORNING						
AFTERNOON						
EVENING						
TOTALS						

MY DAILY ACTIVITY

"Home should be a sanctuary, a place that feels safe and healthy, looks beautiful, and smells wonderful."

—⁊ CHRISTIE MATHESON

We're doing healthy things, eating right, exercising, and getting plenty of sleep. But what about our homes? How can we include our living spaces in our commitment to health?

Creating a healthy home doesn't mean we have to overhaul everything at once. Rather than cleaning out our cupboards in one fell swoop, we can start by incorporating nontoxic and all-natural products as we need them. Obtaining high-quality cleaners, detergents, and soaps—anything that comes into contact with skin or food—reduces our exposure to harmful chemicals and supports our goal of overall well-being.

Today, seek to create a healthy home.

Daily Nutritional Information

Time	Amt.	Cal.	Fat gms	Protein gms	Carbs gms	Fiber gms
MORNING						
AFTERNOON						
EVENING						
TOTALS						

MY DAILY ACTIVITY

_____

_____

_____

_____

_____

_____

_____

_____

_____

_____

> *"It is only possible to live happily ever after on a day-to-day basis."*
>
> — MARGARET BONNANO

Some days we look at our diets or exercise schedules and feel overwhelmed. We can't imagine being able to do this for the rest of our lives. We can't fathom living without our favorite binge food or never having the option to eat whatever we want, whenever we want. We need to remember that we aren't doing this for a lifetime—we're doing it just for today.

Looking at it one day at a time keeps us from getting overwhelmed. Just for today, we can stick to our food plans. Just for today, we can move our bodies. Just for today, we can make the best possible choices for our well-being.

Today, take it one day at a time.

Daily Nutritional Information

Time	Amt.	Cal.	Fat gms	Protein gms	Carbs gms	Fiber gms
MORNING						
AFTERNOON						
EVENING						
TOTALS						

My Daily Activity

_____

_____

_____

_____

_____

_____

_____

_____

_____

_____

> *"Don't wait. The time will never be just right."*
>
> —⍺ NAPOLEON HILL

*I*f we wait until everything else in our lives is perfect before we start taking care of ourselves, we're going to wait a long time. To make lasting, positive change, we need to get into action today, not tomorrow.

Just like as Monday was always the best day to start a diet, tomorrow often seems like the best time to take care of ourselves. Today we're too busy, overwhelmed, overworked, to exercise, eat healthily, or start a spiritual practice. But when *don't* we have obligations and demands on our time?

Today, stop waiting for that magic moment and get moving.

Daily Nutritional Information

Time	Amt.	Cal.	Fat gms	Protein gms	Carbs gms	Fiber gms
MORNING						
AFTERNOON						
EVENING						
TOTALS						

MY DAILY ACTIVITY

> *"Vices are sometimes only virtues carried to excess!"*
>
> —❦ CHARLES DICKENS

There we were, following our plan and feeling great. Next thing we know, we're deep into the bag of chips, box of cookies, or carton of ice cream—and it's empty. What happened? If we've just blown it—and blown it big—what we need is the three-step Binge Recovery Plan:

Step 1. Halt any feelings of shame immediately. Shame is an obstacle that keeps us from moving forward and needlessly wastes our energy.

Step 2. Look at the big picture. What was going on at the time? Were we stressed out, upset, or angry?

Step 3. Ask ourselves what we could have done differently. No experience is wasted if we use it to learn, improve, and continue.

Today, learn from your experiences.

Daily Nutritional Information

Time	Amt.	Cal.	Fat gms	Protein gms	Carbs gms	Fiber gms
MORNING						
AFTERNOON						
EVENING						
TOTALS						

My Daily Activity

_____

_____

_____

_____

_____

_____

_____

_____

_____

"If I buy something new—a piece of clothing, a tie, a shirt, a suit—something old has to go. That's the way I avoid clutter, crammed closets and drawers. It keeps things in balance, and it really works."

—MATT LAUER

*I*f we live in cluttered spaces full of crammed closets and drawers, we're robbing ourselves of the peace of mind and serenity an organized home brings.

No matter how busy we are, we can keep our homes in balance by replacing the old with the new, picking items up off the floor, and putting things away when we're finished with them. With small, consistent actions, we can keep both our minds and homes clutter-free.

Today, do at least one thing to declutter your home.

Daily Nutritional Information

Time	Amt.	Cal.	Fat gms	Protein gms	Carbs gms	Fiber gms
MORNING						
AFTERNOON						
EVENING						
TOTALS						

MY DAILY ACTIVITY

> *"The pessimist sees difficulty in every opportunity. The optimist sees opportunity in every difficulty."*
>
> —⌀ WINSTON CHURCHILL

Cultivating an optimistic outlook is vital to the success of living a healthy life. If we only see the negative—such as the pounds we haven't lost, the test results that haven't changed, or the weights we can't lift—we become discouraged and are tempted to give up.

An optimistic outlook lets us see opportunities for growth in every situation. If the scale hasn't moved in a reasonable amount of time, we may want to increase our fitness by making our exercise routines more challenging. If our test results haven't improved, we may look for more effective treatment. Staying positive keeps us focused on solutions, which keeps us moving forward.

Today, choose optimism.

Daily Nutritional Information

Time	Amt.	Cal.	Fat gms	Protein gms	Carbs gms	Fiber gms
MORNING						
AFTERNOON						
EVENING						
TOTALS						

MY DAILY ACTIVITY

"Dedicate yourself to the good you deserve and desire for yourself. Give yourself peace of mind. You deserve to be happy. You deserve delight."

— MARK VICTOR HANSEN

Come on, you can eat that. You deserve it. When we start hearing the voice in our heads telling us that we deserve to indulge in food that isn't good for us, we need to take a look at what we're really telling ourselves. We may think we're giving ourselves a treat, but we're really setting ourselves up to wallow in regret later. Do we really deserve to do something that may be harmful?

What we deserve are the rewards we get from sticking to our healthy habits, namely, good health and high self-esteem. With a little effort, we can find things other than food to reward ourselves: a good book, a matinee, a nap, a phone call to a friend.

Today, treat yourself in healthy ways.

Daily Nutritional Information

Time	Amt.	Cal.	Fat gms	Protein gms	Carbs gms	Fiber gms
MORNING						
AFTERNOON						
EVENING						
TOTALS						

My Daily Activity

"You know that old joke about the guy who lives to be 104? The punch line goes something like, 'If I knew I was gonna get this old, I'd have taken much better care of myself.' Well, guess what? We actually are living longer, and the time to start taking care of ourselves is right this minute."

— OPRAH WINFREY

*E*ach of us has been given one body in this life, and it's the one we're in right now. We can decorate it, cover it up, or surgically alter it, but it's still our one and only body.

Because we're in lifetime relationships with these bodies of ours, we need to give them the best care we can. Positive, proactive moves like eliminating foods that aren't good for our bodies, taking supplements to support our weak areas, exercising to keep ourselves strong, and resting when we are tired, set the groundwork for a healthy body today and in the future.

Today, make your body your lifelong friend.

Daily Nutritional Information

Time	Amt.	Cal.	Fat gms	Protein gms	Carbs gms	Fiber gms
MORNING						
AFTERNOON						
EVENING						
TOTALS						

MY DAILY ACTIVITY

"Has anybody ever told you, you have a serious impulse control problem?"

—THE RIDDLER TO TWO-FACE, WHO HAS JUST SHOT A HOLE IN THE CEILING OF HIS LAIR. *BATMAN* (1966)

Poor food choices tend to be impulsive—we reach for food as a knee-jerk reaction to uncomfortable situations or feelings. Luckily, we can retrain ourselves to take control of our impulses before we eat.

One powerful impulse-curbing technique is the "thirty-second rule." Pausing and counting to thirty before taking that first bite gives our rational selves time to take over before our impulses kick in. During these thirty seconds, we pause, breathe, and reflect. What's bothering us? What are we feeling? By pausing, we can take control of our impulses, identify what's really going on, and find healthy ways to deal with it other than eating.

Today, use the thirty-second rule.

Daily Nutritional Information

Time	Amt.	Cal.	Fat gms	Protein gms	Carbs gms	Fiber gms
MORNING						
AFTERNOON						
EVENING						
TOTALS						

MY DAILY ACTIVITY

> *"I have gained and lost the same ten pounds so many times over and over again my cellulite must have déjà vu."*
>
> —JANE WAGNER

*M*any of us have spent years as "yo-yo dieters"—going on very-low-calorie diets, rapidly losing weight, then regaining it, plus some. The up-and-down syndrome hurts us not just physically but emotionally, socially, and spiritually as well. We may feel humiliated by our "defeat," embarrassed for people to see us, and hopeless about our situation.

The solution to breaking the yo-yo cycle is to work toward wellness, not weight loss. Rather than having weight loss as the goal, we should focus on exchanging unhealthy habits for healthy ones. This new focus gives us tools not only to lose the weight we want but also to keep it off for good.

Today, say good-bye to yo-yo dieting.

Daily Nutritional Information

Time	Amt.	Cal.	Fat gms	Protein gms	Carbs gms	Fiber gms
MORNING						
AFTERNOON						
EVENING						
TOTALS						

MY DAILY ACTIVITY

_____

_____

_____

_____

_____

_____

_____

_____

_____

"Diet mentality (n): The belief that one can follow a diet until weight loss is achieved and then return to previous eating habits and stay skinny. See also: insanity."

—Anonymous

Wellness isn't about finding a quick fix to lose weight and then returning to old habits; it's about investing in a lifetime of overall health. A program that truly sustains our well-being will easily be incorporated into our lives, support our health goals, and meet our unique emotional, physical, and spiritual needs now and in the future. Anything less is just insanity.

Today, leave the diet mentality behind.

Daily Nutritional Information

Time	Amt.	Cal.	Fat gms	Protein gms	Carbs gms	Fiber gms
MORNING						
AFTERNOON						
EVENING						
TOTALS						

My Daily Activity

> "When the earth is sick and polluted,
> human health is impossible. . . To heal
> ourselves, we must heal our planet,
> and to heal our planet, we must heal
> ourselves."

—◯ BOBBY MCLEOD

We're respecting our emotional, physical, and spiritual selves when we decide to make our lives healthier. Every action we take to improve our lives—whether it's reducing fat in our diets or biking to work—helps our bodies become healthier. Similarly, when we recycle, turn down our thermostats, or pick up litter, we are contributing to a healthier world.

Human actions have caused or increased the impact of many environmental problems we face today—problems that impact the physical health of many of us. In the same way, human actions can help decrease those environmental problems.

Today, respect both your inner and outer worlds.

Daily Nutritional Information

Time	Amt.	Cal.	Fat gms	Protein gms	Carbs gms	Fiber gms
MORNING						
AFTERNOON						
EVENING						
TOTALS						

My Daily Activity

_____

_____

_____

_____

_____

_____

_____

_____

_____

_____

"Breathing correctly is the key to better fitness, muscle strength, stamina and athletic endurance."

—☙ Dr. Michael Yessis

*N*othing is more natural than breathing, which means we may underestimate its power and importance. Done correctly, our breathing can help us reach our fitness goals and can contribute to our emotional and spiritual well-being.

Filling our lungs with oxygen before, during, and after exercise energizes our muscles and aids in their recovery from activity. During the day, we can foster mental clarity and peace of mind by simply sitting quietly, inhaling slowly through the nose, and then exhaling slowly through the mouth, taking six to eight deep breaths per minute. As our diaphragms rise and fall, our minds clear, our bodies relax, and our serenity increases.

Today, just breathe.

Daily Nutritional Information

Time	Amt.	Cal.	Fat gms	Protein gms	Carbs gms	Fiber gms
MORNING						
AFTERNOON						
EVENING						
TOTALS						

MY DAILY ACTIVITY

> *"Seeing is believing."*
>
> —✢ AMERICAN PROVERB

Visual proof is powerful. One tool we can use to keep ourselves motivated and encouraged is a "success collage." Creating a picture of the life we want by clipping images from magazines and then attaching them to a corkboard helps ingrain success into our subconscious minds.

We can put anything we want on our "success collage"—no dream is too big or too small. Maybe we'll choose images of a toned body, a beachside running path, or an organic vegetable garden. Perhaps we'll add a meaningful phrase or two. Keeping our collage in plain view reinforces our goals and the belief that whatever we dream, we can achieve.

Today, make a "success collage."

Daily Nutritional Information

Time	Amt.	Cal.	Fat gms	Protein gms	Carbs gms	Fiber gms
MORNING						
AFTERNOON						
EVENING						
TOTALS						

MY DAILY ACTIVITY

_____

_____

_____

_____

_____

_____

_____

_____

_____

> *"A journey of a thousand sites begins with a single click."*
>
> —⌁ ANONYMOUS

*I*magine what we could accomplish if we tapped into the strength and experience of a vast network of people who shared our goal of achieving optimum health? That network is a reality—the Internet.

With a few clicks of a mouse, we can connect to an online community and benefit from the experience and real-world advice of people we would not otherwise meet. A quick online search will find multiple Web sites where we can do everything from creating personal profiles to swapping tips on workout techniques, recipes, and positive thinking. Joining a large supportive community reinforces our programs and reminds us we're all in this together.

Today, tap into the power of an online community.

Daily Nutritional Information

Time	Amt.	Cal.	Fat gms	Protein gms	Carbs gms	Fiber gms
MORNING						
AFTERNOON						
EVENING						
TOTALS						

MY DAILY ACTIVITY

"Have patience with all things, but chiefly have patience with yourself. Do not lose courage in considering your own imperfections but instantly set about remedying them—every day begin the task anew."

—SAINT FRANCIS DE SALES

The road to wellness is a journey most of us travel imperfectly. It is a rare traveler who doesn't at times veer off the path, take a sudden detour, or stop dead in the middle of the road.

If we're off-track, it's essential that we remedy our course right away. With patience and persistence, we can get moving again. We must never lose courage and we must never stop our journey before we get to our final destination—total health, wellness, and happiness.

Today, keep moving forward.

Daily Nutritional Information

Time	Amt.	Cal.	Fat gms	Protein gms	Carbs gms	Fiber gms
MORNING						
AFTERNOON						
EVENING						
TOTALS						

MY DAILY ACTIVITY

_____

_____

_____

_____

_____

_____

_____

_____

_____

> *"Bring the body and the mind will follow."*
>
> — AMERICAN SAYING

W hat do we do on those days when we'd rather curl up on the couch with a good book than exercise? Sometimes we have to trust that if we get ourselves up and moving, we'll find ourselves getting engaged in and enjoying activity.

Typically, getting started is the hardest part during a low-motivation day. If we can just get moving, our bodies will take over and release the feel-good endorphins that give us energy and stamina. When we're done, we will feel better both physically and about ourselves.

Today, move your body and trust your mind will follow.

Daily Nutritional Information

Time	Amt.	Cal.	Fat gms	Protein gms	Carbs gms	Fiber gms
MORNING						
AFTERNOON						
EVENING						
TOTALS						

My Daily Activity

_____

_____

_____

_____

_____

_____

_____

_____

_____

> *"To be a consistent winner means preparing for not just one day, one month or even one year—but for a lifetime."*
>
> —BILL RODGERS

If getting healthier were an Olympic sport, it would be a marathon, not a fifty-yard dash. The successful runners are those who take a long-term focus on creating overall health, not a short-term focus on losing weight.

The best way to run the wellness marathon is to train for life. We can look at daily, weekly, and monthly goals as races and the year as a season. If we prepare long term, we can effectively manage our time, focus, food, and exercise. With a marathon perspective, we can be confident knowing we can win the weight-loss race and that we will also cross the finish line to wellness.

Today, be a marathon runner, not a sprinter.

Daily Nutritional Information

Time	Amt.	Cal.	Fat gms	Protein gms	Carbs gms	Fiber gms
MORNING						
AFTERNOON						
EVENING						
TOTALS						

MY DAILY ACTIVITY

> " 'Tis not the meat, but 'tis the
> appetite makes eating a delight."
>
> —John Suckling

*H*ow many of us have spent lifetimes believing that if we could just control our appetites, we could control how our bodies looked? We may have subjected ourselves to unhealthy appetite-suppressant methods such as unbalanced diets, caffeine, nicotine, pills. In truth, we look and feel our best when we work with, not against, our appetites.

Physical hunger is the language our bodies use to tell us what they need. If we listen, we'll learn how to feed them, what and how much they need, and when they need it. When we stop fighting our appetites and think of them as communications from our bodies, we can properly nourish ourselves and become strong, lean, and healthy.

Today, listen to your appetite.

Daily Nutritional Information

Time	Amt.	Cal.	Fat gms	Protein gms	Carbs gms	Fiber gms
MORNING						
AFTERNOON						
EVENING						
TOTALS						

My Daily Activity

_____

_____

_____

_____

_____

_____

_____

_____

_____

> "While we may not be able to control all that happens to us, we can control what happens inside."
>
> — ᗡ BENJAMIN FRANKLIN

*D*eadlines, distractions, and demands can make it difficult to focus on our health, and we can easily find ourselves grabbing fast but unhealthy food to make it through the day. The solution is to take charge of our schedules and make taking care of ourselves as much a priority as our careers.

Ironically, prioritizing our food and exercise habits won't just make us healthier and happier, it also will improve the quality of our work. When we eat high-sugar, low-quality food, we get an immediate boost, but we are likely to end up feeling sluggish and drained at the end of the day. When we fuel up right, we can work with more energy, productivity, and confidence.

Today, treat your health like a career.

Daily Nutritional Information

Time	Amt.	Cal.	Fat gms	Protein gms	Carbs gms	Fiber gms
MORNING						
AFTERNOON						
EVENING						
TOTALS						

MY DAILY ACTIVITY

> *"Keep your face always toward the sunshine—and shadows will fall behind you."*
>
> —❧ WALT WHITMAN

a healthy dose of carefully monitored sunshine can bring about a multitude of physical and emotional benefits.

Sunshine enhances our emotional stability by stimulating the production of the feel-good neurotransmitter serotonin, which promotes a positive outlook and fights depression. We get 90 percent of our vitamin D through sunshine, and it helps our bodies produce the hormone melatonin, which helps regulate sleep and wake cycles. A little sun can go a long way to brighten our lives.

Today, enjoy the sunshine.

Daily Nutritional Information

Time	Amt.	Cal.	Fat gms	Protein gms	Carbs gms	Fiber gms
MORNING						
AFTERNOON						
EVENING						
TOTALS						

My Daily Activity

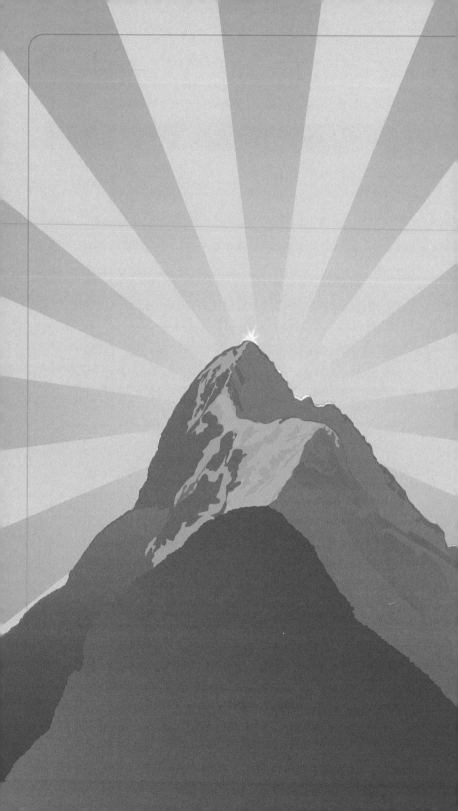

Overcome Obstacles

"Curious things, habits. People themselves never knew they had them."

—&c AGATHA CHRISTIE

*a*wareness is the first step in changing a habit. Once we know we have a habit, we can do what we need to change it.

If we discover that we head back into the kitchen late at night, for example, we can create other, healthier habits such as finding night-owl friends to call or even going to bed earlier. Understanding old habits that don't work lets us replace them with new ones that do. When we change our habits, we change our lives.

Today, be aware of your habits.

Daily Nutritional Information

Time	Amt.	Cal.	Fat gms	Protein gms	Carbs gms	Fiber gms
MORNING						
AFTERNOON						
EVENING						
TOTALS						

MY DAILY ACTIVITY

_____

_____

_____

_____

_____

_____

_____

_____

_____

> *"Deciding to commit yourself to long-term results, rather than short-term fixes, is as important as any decision you'll make in your lifetime."*
>
> —Tony Robbins

We cut carbs for the class reunion, join a gym for swimsuit season, or forget fast food to get our bad cholesterol down. Goal setting is a worthy venture, but if we set health goals for specific events, when they're over, we tend to lose our motivation and go back to old, unhealthy habits.

For lasting results, we need to put our calendars away and approach health as a holistic, lifetime commitment to total well-being. When we change our attitude from a quick fix to a lifelong perspective, ironically, we can look and feel our best at any event we attend.

Today, trade in your short-term goals for long-term well-being.

Daily Nutritional Information

Time	Amt.	Cal.	Fat gms	Protein gms	Carbs gms	Fiber gms
MORNING						
AFTERNOON						
EVENING						
TOTALS						

MY DAILY ACTIVITY

_____
_____
_____
_____
_____
_____
_____
_____
_____

"Each body has its art."

— GWENDOLYN BROOKS

*S*ome days we look in the mirror and don't like anything we see. We don't like our legs. We hate our arms. We really hate our stomachs. The constant stream of this kind of self-criticism is painful as we do it and erodes our self-esteem.

On days when nothing about us seems right, we need to switch from negative to positive thinking. Instead of berating our bodies, we can cultivate appreciation for their remarkable resilience, strength, and ability to rejuvenate. We can view our bodies' idiosyncrasies, scars, and quirks as a living diary of where we've been and what we've survived. With a new perspective, we'll be able to look in the mirror and appreciate our bodies' unique art.

Today, start to appreciate your body.

Daily Nutritional Information

Time	Amt.	Cal.	Fat gms	Protein gms	Carbs gms	Fiber gms
MORNING						
AFTERNOON						
EVENING						
TOTALS						

MY DAILY ACTIVITY

_____

_____

_____

_____

_____

_____

_____

_____

_____

_____

> *"Meditate daily, and soon your inner strength and mind power will grow."*
>
> —⟳ REMEZ SASSON

M editation is an ancient practice that brings modern-day peace of mind. Once thought to be the exclusive and mysterious skill of ancient yogis, meditation is an effective and healthy way to battle stress, encourage emotional balance, and revitalize energy.

If we're new to meditating, we can start by sitting quietly and focusing on our breathing, which relaxes us both mentally and physically. If we're experienced, we can expand our practice and learn to incorporate more advanced meditation principles into everyday living. No matter how we do it or how much we do, we benefit physically, emotionally, and spiritually when we take time to meditate.

Today, meditate.

Daily Nutritional Information

Time	Amt.	Cal.	Fat gms	Protein gms	Carbs gms	Fiber gms
MORNING						
AFTERNOON						
EVENING						
TOTALS						

MY DAILY ACTIVITY

_____

_____

_____

_____

_____

_____

_____

_____

_____

> "A good stance and posture reflect a proper state of mind."
>
> —🖋 MORIHEI UESHIBA

a single, simple thing can immediately improve our appearance, health, and attitude: good old-fashioned posture. Standing up straight with shoulders back and neck aligned makes us instantly taller and thinner, puts our spines in their proper alignment, and evokes a sense of self-confidence.

Not only do we get instant physical and emotional benefits, we get future ones as well. When we allow our spines to slouch, we cause strain on our neck and shoulder muscles, making us more prone to injury. Pulling our shoulders back, standing tall, and looking the world in the eye keeps us looking up and feeling great, now and later.

Today, stand up straight.

Daily Nutritional Information

Time	Amt.	Cal.	Fat gms	Protein gms	Carbs gms	Fiber gms
MORNING						
AFTERNOON						
EVENING						
TOTALS						

My Daily Activity

_____

_____

_____

_____

_____

_____

_____

_____

_____

"Fad diets are just that. Rapid weight loss leads to equally rapid weight gain. There's no evidence that fad diets are effective in long term. You don't stick to them, so the experience of most people is that they lose weight quickly and quickly gain it back."

—JIM DAVIS

As tempting as it may be to jump-start weight loss with a fad diet, we need to remember that weight loss isn't the goal—wellness is. When considering a diet, we need to ask ourselves if it's a plan that will serve our bodies, lifestyles, and budgets for the long haul. Then we need to check in with our healthcare provider and get a professional's approval.

By taking good care of ourselves, we will not only lose the weight we want, we'll gain long-term health and peace of mind.

Today, choose long-term wellness.

Daily Nutritional Information

Time	Amt.	Cal.	Fat gms	Protein gms	Carbs gms	Fiber gms
MORNING						
AFTERNOON						
EVENING						
TOTALS						

MY DAILY ACTIVITY

_____

_____

_____

_____

_____

_____

_____

_____

_____

_____

"Tell your wife that she looks pretty, even if she looks like a truck hit her."

—Ricky, age 10, when asked how to make a marriage work

Compliments tend to come to us when we're taking care of ourselves. We look great, we feel great, and people notice our looser clothes and positive attitudes. It's the times we look and feel like a truck hit us that we need compliments the most. This is also the time we may not get them. Rather than waiting to receive a compliment, why not give one?

Is there someone in the office who looks stressed? We can find something she or he did well and say so. Does our waitress look frazzled? We can thank her for doing a great job. Giving joy brings joy. We get the very boost we need by giving it to others.

Today, compliment someone who seems to need it.

Daily Nutritional Information

Time	Amt.	Cal.	Fat gms	Protein gms	Carbs gms	Fiber gms
MORNING						
AFTERNOON						
EVENING						
TOTALS						

My Daily Activity

_____

_____

_____

_____

_____

_____

_____

_____

_____

> *"Life is a great and wondrous mystery, and the only thing we know that we have for sure is what is right here right now. Don't miss it."*
>
> —⟶ LEO BUSCAGLIA

Most of us spend our days with our bodies in one place and our minds in another. We're eating breakfast but reading the paper or ruminating about what happened at work yesterday. We're eating dinner but watching TV or planning what we need to do tomorrow. Thinking too much about yesterday or tomorrow robs us of what's right in front of us: today.

We can start becoming present to our lives by first becoming aware of what we're eating. Giving meals our full attention allows us to recognize how our bodies feel. Being connected with our bodies focuses our minds on what's going on right here, right now, today.

Today, don't miss today.

Daily Nutritional Information

Time	Amt.	Cal.	Fat gms	Protein gms	Carbs gms	Fiber gms
MORNING						
AFTERNOON						
EVENING						
TOTALS						

MY DAILY ACTIVITY

> *"Health is a state of complete physical, mental, and social well-being, and not merely the absence of disease or infirmity."*
>
> — WORLD HEALTH ORGANIZATION, 1948

Why wait until we get sick to get well? Becoming an advocate for our own health maximizes our chances of living long, healthy, and productive lives. We can take steps now to prevent illness, aches, or pains in the future that result from not taking care of ourselves.

What if we are already ill in some way? All the more reason to give ourselves the best care available. Nothing is more healing to a weak system than good food, exercise, fresh air and sunshine, hydration, and peace of mind.

Today, be your own health advocate.

Daily Nutritional Information

Time	Amt.	Cal.	Fat gms	Protein gms	Carbs gms	Fiber gms
MORNING						
AFTERNOON						
EVENING						
TOTALS						

MY DAILY ACTIVITY

_____

_____

_____

_____

_____

_____

_____

_____

_____

"It's not a successful climb unless you enjoy the journey."

—DAN BENSON

We can and should stay focused on our goals, but not at the expense of the journey. Appreciating the small victories along the way—our improved strength, the looser clothes, our increased peace of mind—ensures we don't miss the most important part of any process: the lessons we learn getting there.

Today, make sure to enjoy the road.

Daily Nutritional Information

Time	Amt.	Cal.	Fat gms	Protein gms	Carbs gms	Fiber gms
MORNING						
AFTERNOON						
EVENING						
TOTALS						

MY DAILY ACTIVITY

_____

_____

_____

_____

_____

_____

_____

_____

_____

"The dying process begins the minute we are born, but it accelerates during dinner parties."

—CAROL MATTHAU

Like it or not, parties happen. For a person on a special food plan, parties can be very anxiety producing. We can worry about the food that's being served and whether there will be anything we can eat. The key to peace of mind when attending any get-together—whether it's an office function, wedding, or holiday party—is preparation.

With every invitation come options. We can call ahead and ask what's being served and offer to help the host by bringing a dish. We can decide to eat before or after. Potlucks are easy— we bring food we can eat and enough to share. Well prepared, we can stop worrying about the food and have fun instead.

Today, party with confidence.

Daily Nutritional Information

Time	Amt.	Cal.	Fat gms	Protein gms	Carbs gms	Fiber gms
MORNING						
AFTERNOON						
EVENING						
TOTALS						

MY DAILY ACTIVITY

_____

_____

_____

_____

_____

_____

_____

_____

_____

> *"It's not stress that kills us, it is our reaction to it."*
>
> —HANS SELYE

Many of us use food as a stress-management tool. We get overwhelmed and head right for the comfort food. Stress is a part of life, so how can we cope without eating? As tempting as it is to have a mini-breakdown or to binge under pressure, we need to train ourselves to stay calm and focused—and to maintain healthy eating.

We can learn healthy coping tools. Instead of diving into the refrigerator, we can breathe, close our eyes for a moment, then regroup. Maybe we can physically step away from the task at hand and get some air. Perhaps we can ask someone for help. Every challenge we face without eating for relief builds not only our coping muscles but also our self-esteem and confidence.

Today, use healthy tools to handle stress.

Daily Nutritional Information

Time	Amt.	Cal.	Fat gms	Protein gms	Carbs gms	Fiber gms
MORNING						
AFTERNOON						
EVENING						
TOTALS						

My Daily Activity

_____

_____

_____

_____

_____

_____

_____

_____

_____

> *"Every survival kit should include a sense of humor."*
>
> —⟲ ANONYMOUS

*I*f laughter is the best medicine, why do we abandon our sense of humor as soon as we start a fitness program? We may be unhappy about having to give up unhealthy foods. We may dislike exercise. A little humor can go a long way toward making difficult tasks easier.

We need to take our health seriously, but not ourselves. When we admit and joke about our struggles rather than suffer in silence, not only do we lighten our loads, we may even discover others feel the same way. Then we can all laugh together.

Today, keep your sense of humor.

Daily Nutritional Information

Time	Amt.	Cal.	Fat gms	Protein gms	Carbs gms	Fiber gms
MORNING						
AFTERNOON						
EVENING						
TOTALS						

MY DAILY ACTIVITY

> *"You have to expect things of yourself before you can do them."*
>
> —<small>MICHAEL JORDAN</small>

When we committed to getting and staying fit, we did more than just commit to healthy eating, exercise, and good habits—we made promises to ourselves. Promises to invest in the longevity of our bodies, break self-destructive patterns, become our best selves. Yet, we live in the real world, and temptation to eat what we shouldn't or to avoid exercise is everywhere. How can we find the strength to keep those promises?

One simple question can save our sanity: *Is it worth it?* Is it worth it to eat something that will compromise our health and self-esteem? Is it worth it to jeopardize our progress? Pausing to consider the consequences of poor choices allows us to see the big picture. Connected to the truth, we are more likely to stay committed to fulfilling our promises to ourselves.

Today, remain true to yourself.

Daily Nutritional Information

Time	Amt.	Cal.	Fat gms	Protein gms	Carbs gms	Fiber gms
MORNING						
AFTERNOON						
EVENING						
TOTALS						

MY DAILY ACTIVITY

"Focus on your problem zones, your strength, your energy, your flexibility and all the rest. Also, you should change your program every thirty days. That's the key."

—JACK LALANNE

*C*hange is the one constant we all need in our exercise routines. Shaking up our routines keeps us at our best by challenging our strength, flexibility, and endurance.

Changing our routines also shakes up our minds. New activities may lead us to discover strengths, preferences, and talents we never knew we had. A dance class may show us we have a natural rhythm. Or we may uncover a reserve of core strength during a yoga class. When it comes to exercise, variety is the spice of life.

Today, change it up.

Daily Nutritional Information

Time	Amt.	Cal.	Fat gms	Protein gms	Carbs gms	Fiber gms
MORNING						
AFTERNOON						
EVENING						
TOTALS						

My Daily Activity

_____

_____

_____

_____

_____

_____

_____

_____

_____

_____

> *"The best number for a dinner party is two: myself and a good head waiter."*
>
> —⌒ NUBAR GULBENKIAN

*H*ow many times have we heard—or said—that eating in restaurants makes it impossible to eat healthy, balanced meals? In truth, with a little effort, restaurant dining can be both satisfying and healthy.

A key ingredient to restaurant success is making friends with the food server. Asking specific questions about a meal enables us to make substitutions and adjustments to take care of ourselves. How many ounces are in the main dish? Does the sauce have sugar in it? The server can also help us by talking to the chef, suggesting entrées, or even requesting a special meal for us. Eating well in restaurants is possible—with a little help from our friends.

Today, make dining out a healthy experience.

Daily Nutritional Information

Time	Amt.	Cal.	Fat gms	Protein gms	Carbs gms	Fiber gms
MORNING						
AFTERNOON						
EVENING						
TOTALS						

My Daily Activity

"I try to do one new thing every day—if it's picking up a book by an unfamiliar author or even sitting in a different chair with my morning coffee, if only to see my house from a fresh perspective to keep the mind alert and alive."

—LETTY COTTIN POGREBIN

Keeping our minds alert and engaged is essential to living in a healthy way. The human brain remains fluid throughout life, restructuring itself according to what it learns. If we stay in the same routine, day after day, year after year, we are literally locking our minds into gridlock.

Getting mentally unstuck is easier than we think; it is only a matter of "shaking up our brains" by engaging in activities that are unfamiliar. It can be as simple as driving a different way to work, using the nonprimary hand to eat, or revamping our hairstyle. When we shake things up, we get a fresh perspective.

Today, think of one thing you can do to shake up your brain.

Daily Nutritional Information

Time	Amt.	Cal.	Fat gms	Protein gms	Carbs gms	Fiber gms
MORNING						
AFTERNOON						
EVENING						
TOTALS						

My Daily Activity

> *"Feed your skin from within with a choice of appropriate foods to keep it looking clear, healthy, and radiant."*
>
> —⌒ VASU NARGUNDKAR

*H*ealthy skin is about more than just good looks; it's essential to good health. Our skin is our largest organ and it protects us from the elements, which means we have to take care of it so that it can function at its best for a lifetime.

Proper skincare doesn't have to be time-consuming or expensive. The best way to care for our skin is to live healthy lifestyles. Proper nutrition and hydration, regular exercise, and adequate sleep show up positively on our skin. We can build on those good health habits with a daily routine that includes cleansing, moisturizing, using sunscreen, and getting regular checkups.

Today, be good to your skin.

Daily Nutritional Information

Time	Amt.	Cal.	Fat gms	Protein gms	Carbs gms	Fiber gms
MORNING						
AFTERNOON						
EVENING						
TOTALS						

My Daily Activity

> "Honor begets honor; trust begets trust; faith begets faith; and hope is the mainspring of life."
>
> —Henry L. Stimson

Most of us are familiar with momentum in a negative sense. If we've fallen off our healthy routines, it's easier for us to then skip exercise, which makes it easier for us to eat poorly tomorrow. But momentum also works in reverse: We can build positive momentum.

The more positive changes and actions we take, the more we pave the way for even more positive changes and action. For example, if we work out, we feel good, which motivates us to eat better. The more positive action we do, the more positive action we do.

Today, create a positive momentum.

Daily Nutritional Information

Time	Amt.	Cal.	Fat gms	Protein gms	Carbs gms	Fiber gms
MORNING						
AFTERNOON						
EVENING						
TOTALS						

My Daily Activity

_____

_____

_____

_____

_____

_____

_____

_____

_____

Who doesn't look back on her life and wish she'd made different choices? It's easy to waste an enormous amount of time torturing ourselves with "what if?" What if I had taken better care of my body? What if I had taken that other job? What if I hadn't wasted years in that terrible relationship?

"What if?" paralyzes us. To move forward, we need to change the question from "What if?" to "What can I do now?" What can I do now to improve my health? What can I do now to make my current job better? What can I do now to learn from my past decisions and move forward?

Today, change "What if?" to "What can I do now?"

Daily Nutritional Information

Time	Amt.	Cal.	Fat gms	Protein gms	Carbs gms	Fiber gms
MORNING						
AFTERNOON						
EVENING						
TOTALS						

My Daily Activity

_____

_____

_____

_____

_____

_____

_____

_____

_____

_____

"Humor is a rubber sword—it allows you to make a point without drawing blood."

—MARY HIRSCH

We are surrounded: Negative and difficult people are everywhere. Sometimes they're our neighbors and sometimes they're working in the next cubicle. We can easily find ourselves battling the embittered. For those of us with tendencies to lick spoonfuls of ice cream along with our wounds, finding healthy ways to defend ourselves from problematic people can be challenging. We have one powerful guerrilla tactic we can deploy: humor.

In tense situations, a strategically placed joke can diffuse anger and pave the way to a mature discussion. At other times, putting a positive spin on a negative comment can lead the conversation in a new, more productive direction. Whatever our tactic, a little humor can make the difference between war and peace.

Today, arm yourself with humor.

Daily Nutritional Information

Time	Amt.	Cal.	Fat gms	Protein gms	Carbs gms	Fiber gms
MORNING						
AFTERNOON						
EVENING						
TOTALS						

MY DAILY ACTIVITY

> *"Success comes in cans, not can't's."*
>
> —֍ ANONYMOUS

S witching "can't" to "can" is crucial to wellness. Perhaps we think we can't get healthy until we have more support at home. Perhaps we believe we can't eat healthy meals in restaurants or while traveling. Or, we feel we can't possibly follow our exercise routine for one more day.

We can get healthy regardless of anyone or anything. We can eat healthily in restaurants and yes, we can exercise for one more day.

Today, notice when you tell yourself you can't—and then decide you can.

Daily Nutritional Information

Time	Amt.	Cal.	Fat gms	Protein gms	Carbs gms	Fiber gms
MORNING						
AFTERNOON						
EVENING						
TOTALS						

MY DAILY ACTIVITY

"People say that losing weight is no walk in the park. When I hear that, I think, yeah, that's the problem."

—CHRIS ADAMS

Getting fit isn't necessarily easy, but it may not be as difficult as we sometimes make it. Adding a regular, pleasurable walk into our daily routines can make a dramatic difference in how we feel, look, and function.

A walk—around the block, up the stairs, from the far side of the parking lot—is easy to fit into our routines. Even if we did nothing else to become healthier, adding a walk of ten, twenty, or thirty minutes or more to our activity each day can significantly improve our health.

Today, take a walk.

Daily Nutritional Information

Time	Amt.	Cal.	Fat gms	Protein gms	Carbs gms	Fiber gms
MORNING						
AFTERNOON						
EVENING						
TOTALS						

MY DAILY ACTIVITY

> *"The body says what words cannot."*
>
> —◦ MARTHA GRAHAM

Our bodies never lie; they tell the truth about who we are and what we're feeling. Every gesture, movement, and stance communicates how we feel. When our self-esteem is low, we tend to hunch our shoulders, avoid eye contact, and cross our arms. When we're feeling good, we look people in the eye, pull our shoulders back, and relax our arms.

Because of the mind–body connection, we can improve our moods by deliberately improving our body language. When we don't feel at our best, we can stand up straight and act as if we feel good. Our minds will eventually catch up and soon our good mood will be genuine.

Today, choose positive body language.

Daily Nutritional Information

Time	Amt.	Cal.	Fat gms	Protein gms	Carbs gms	Fiber gms
MORNING						
AFTERNOON						
EVENING						
TOTALS						

MY DAILY ACTIVITY

"Pleasure, or slow eating, is about savoring every bite that you take. And, so, . . . it's really enjoying the food, really making it a holistic experience."

—LISA DORFMAN

*M*any of us have spent so many years vacillating between dieting and overeating that we no longer recognize when we're hungry before we eat or comfortably full after. We needn't worry; we can regain our connection to our bodies by simply paying attention.

Slow, mindful eating is how we learn what our bodies need. When we sit down to eat, we can take our time and concentrate on really tasting our food. We can feel when our bodies have had enough; then we can put down our forks, feeling satisfied and comfortable.

Today, when you are eating, tune in to your body's signals.

Daily Nutritional Information

Time	Amt.	Cal.	Fat gms	Protein gms	Carbs gms	Fiber gms
MORNING						
AFTERNOON						
EVENING						
TOTALS						

MY DAILY ACTIVITY

"Diet Rule #1: If you eat something and no one sees you eat it, it has no calories."

—Anonymous

Some diet rules are based in fact and some are not. Take the No Second Helpings Rule. It's not necessarily true that we can lose weight by limiting ourselves to a single plate of food at a meal . . . especially if we believe in the Always Clean Your Plate Rule. If we have only one shot at eating—and we have to eat everything on our plates—it makes sense that we'd be more likely to pile food on our plates and eat every bite.

Now is the time to uncover, discover, and discard any old, ingrained diet rules that don't work for us. We get to make our own diet rules—or no rules at all. It's between us and our bodies.

Today, reevaluate your diet rules.

Daily Nutritional Information

Time	Amt.	Cal.	Fat gms	Protein gms	Carbs gms	Fiber gms
MORNING						
AFTERNOON						
EVENING						
TOTALS						

My Daily Activity

_____

_____

_____

_____

_____

_____

_____

_____

_____

_____

"Never eat more than you can lift."

—😊 MISS PIGGY

*D*on't eat after sundown. Don't eat anything that can look back at us. Don't eat anything processed. The list of diet rules goes on and on, full of "don'ts," "shouldn'ts," and "have tos." We may lose a few pounds restricting our food choices according to one of these rules, but, ultimately, following unbalanced diets risks our long-term health and well-being.

To be physically and emotionally fit for the long term, we need to stick to reasonable, well-balanced diets that focus on the healthy food we can eat, not on a list of diet "don'ts."

Today, write down the diet rules that no longer serve you.

Daily Nutritional Information

Time	Amt.	Cal.	Fat gms	Protein gms	Carbs gms	Fiber gms
MORNING						
AFTERNOON						
EVENING						
TOTALS						

My Daily Activity

> *"Once you replace negative thoughts with positive ones, you'll start having positive results."*
>
> —Willie Nelson

*T*his is too hard. I can't do this. What's the use? We all experience negative thoughts at times, especially when we're feeling discouraged or frustrated. For those of us working to live a healthier life, allowing too much negativity can lead to slipping back into unhealthy behavior. As difficult as it can be at times, we need to practice replacing negative thoughts for positive ones.

Just as with any skill, the more we practice positive thinking, the stronger it becomes and the weaker negative thoughts become. Our efforts will pay off in renewed enthusiasm, hope, and energy.

Today, practice positive thinking.

Daily Nutritional Information

Time	Amt.	Cal.	Fat gms	Protein gms	Carbs gms	Fiber gms
MORNING						
AFTERNOON						
EVENING						
TOTALS						

MY DAILY ACTIVITY

_____

_____

_____

_____

_____

_____

_____

_____

> *"In preparing for battle I have always found that plans are useless, but planning is indispensable."*
>
> — DWIGHT D. EISENHOWER

Most of us have at least one time during the day when our willpower wanes. Some of us crave the quick pick-me-up of a sugary snack during a long afternoon. Others tend to collapse after a tough day, TV remote in one hand, binge food in the other. Once we identify our weak moments, we can prepare for them.

Would an afternoon break help us make it through the afternoon without eating? After a hard day, can we talk with a supportive friend or squeeze in a quick fifteen minutes of exercise? Planning ahead will give us strength to successfully stick to our healthy goals.

Today, identify your weak moments and plan what you can do to take care of yourself.

Daily Nutritional Information

Time	Amt.	Cal.	Fat gms	Protein gms	Carbs gms	Fiber gms
MORNING						
AFTERNOON						
EVENING						
TOTALS						

MY DAILY ACTIVITY

"I have to exercise in the morning before my brain figures out what I'm doing."

—◌ MARSHA DOBLE

When we have established healthy routines, we can follow them without having to argue ourselves into—or out of—them. If we let ourselves "negotiate" over whether to eat healthy food (we can eat whatever we want tonight; we'll make up for it tomorrow) or exercise (we're sure that we got enough exercise just cleaning the house; we don't have to go to the gym today), we're bound to lose the negotiation at least some of the time.

It's better if we just do what we need to, without considering other possible options—especially when the options include putting off what we know we need to do.

Today, just do it.

Daily Nutritional Information

Time	Amt.	Cal.	Fat gms	Protein gms	Carbs gms	Fiber gms
MORNING						
AFTERNOON						
EVENING						
TOTALS						

My Daily Activity

> *"Health is a large word. It embraces not the body only, but the mind and spirit as well."*
>
> —James H. West

We may be so impatient to see results that we end up doing things that, ironically, stall our progress. To lose weight more quickly, for example, we may start skipping meals, which sets us up to binge late at night because we feel like we're starving. We injure ourselves by lifting weights that are far too heavy for us in an attempt to get stronger, faster.

We need perspective. Specific goals are just parts of wellness efforts that address our entire selves—emotional, physical, and spiritual. Remembering that we are working to improve our overall health—not just meet specific goals—will help keep our impatience at bay and our progress steady.

Today, look at the big picture.

Daily Nutritional Information

Time	Amt.	Cal.	Fat gms	Protein gms	Carbs gms	Fiber gms
MORNING						
AFTERNOON						
EVENING						
TOTALS						

My Daily Activity

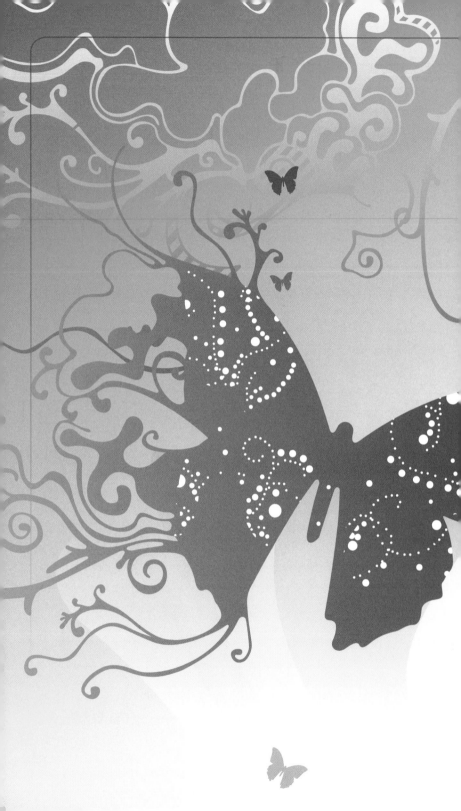

Month 4

Embrace Change

"Ask not what you can do for your country. Ask what's for lunch."

—ɔ ORSON WELLES

*I*f we haven't packed our lunch since grade school, we may want to pick up this old habit again. Not only have brown paper bags morphed into multicompartment, temperature-controlling food containers, but packing a lunch also is an excellent way to keep healthy eating on track, save money, and prevent leftovers from going to waste in the back of the refrigerator.

When we pack our own lunch, we can control portions and know exactly what's in the food we're eating. Homemade lunches free up our time: If we don't have to wait in line or search for a restaurant, we can eat in the quiet of a nearby park or with a friend.

Today, break out the brown bag.

Daily Nutritional Information

Time	Amt.	Cal.	Fat gms	Protein gms	Carbs gms	Fiber gms
MORNING						
AFTERNOON						
EVENING						
TOTALS						

My Daily Activity

_____

_____

_____

_____

_____

_____

_____

_____

_____

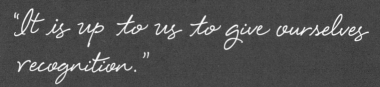

"It is up to us to give ourselves recognition."

—⌁ SPENCER TRACY

We're working hard toward fitness, eating right and exercising—we deserve a treat, right? Absolutely! We keep our drive alive by making sure we reward ourselves for our efforts. The trick is to discover ways to treat ourselves that are also good for us.

What can we indulge in that will make us feel good? Download a favorite tune? Get our nails done? Sleep until noon? Pairing hard work with deserved pampering keeps us motivated and working toward our goals.

Today, reward your hard work.

Daily Nutritional Information

Time	Amt.	Cal.	Fat gms	Protein gms	Carbs gms	Fiber gms
MORNING						
AFTERNOON						
EVENING						
TOTALS						

MY DAILY ACTIVITY

_____

_____

_____

_____

_____

_____

_____

_____

_____

> *"Who is rich? He who rejoices in his portion."*
>
> — THE TALMUD

Wouldn't it be nice if we had all the money in the world to eat the healthiest food we could find and to have the best trainers and equipment at our disposal? Fortunately, we don't have to be rich to be healthy—it's possible to take care of both our bodies and our budgets.

Healthful eating doesn't necessarily mean sticking only with high-end food; we can stock up on inexpensive canned and frozen produce and protein. We can buy organic food at farmers' markets, stockpile during sales, save money using coupons. With some effort and creativity, we can create a healthy food plan using satisfying, affordable food. Exercise can be as simple as a walk around the neighborhood, stretches in our own living room, and using cans of food as weights for strength training.

Today, be a fitness bargain hunter.

Daily Nutritional Information

Time	Amt.	Cal.	Fat gms	Protein gms	Carbs gms	Fiber gms
MORNING						
AFTERNOON						
EVENING						
TOTALS						

My Daily Activity

"A man, ninety years old, was asked to what he attributed his longevity. I reckon, he said, with a twinkle in his eye, it is because most nights I went to bed and slept when I should have sat up and worried."

—⟂ GARSON KANIN

Worrying and eating often go hand in hand; the more worried we feel, the more carelessly we eat. Rather than soothing ourselves with food, we can learn to rein in our worries and find real solutions to what's bothering us.

Whether we're fretting about finances, kids, or the state of the nation, the first step to being worry-free is to list our fears on paper. Seeing them in black and white removes their power and gives us the clarity to come up with feasible solutions. The next step is to take positive, constructive action. Once we get moving, life will feel more manageable and we'll feel calmer. The calmer we feel, the less we look to food for comfort.

Today, write your worries away.

Daily Nutritional Information

Time	Amt.	Cal.	Fat gms	Protein gms	Carbs gms	Fiber gms
MORNING						
AFTERNOON						
EVENING						
TOTALS						

MY DAILY ACTIVITY

_____

_____

_____

_____

_____

_____

_____

_____

> *"I have a hobby . . . I have the world's largest collection of seashells. I keep it scattered on beaches all over the world. Maybe you've seen some of it."*
>
> —Steven Wright

"So, do you have any hobbies?" A deceptively simple question, this can be one of the most difficult to answer. For many of us, eating was our hobby. Although we still love to eat, now that we're eating less for recreation and more for nourishment, it's time to figure out what else we like to do.

A little introspection is a good start. If money and time weren't an issue, what would we really like to do? Do we love art, fabric, photographs, building things? Once we identify our interests, we can develop meaningful and perhaps even lifelong hobbies around them.

Today, find a new hobby.

Daily Nutritional Information

Time	Amt.	Cal.	Fat gms	Protein gms	Carbs gms	Fiber gms
MORNING						
AFTERNOON						
EVENING						
TOTALS						

MY DAILY ACTIVITY

"Fall down seven times, get up eight."

*G*etting to the fitness level we want can be a series of taking two steps forward and one step back. The biggest mistake we can make if we've fallen off our goals is to get discouraged, stay on the floor, and not get up.

Slips contain valuable lessons that can make us stronger in the long run. If we slip, instead of beating ourselves up with needless guilt, we can review what happened and use that information to make better choices next time. When we use our slips as opportunities to learn, we can be assured that, no matter how many times we fall, we'll be walking in no time.

Today, if you fall down, get up and keep walking.

Daily Nutritional Information

Time	Amt.	Cal.	Fat gms	Protein gms	Carbs gms	Fiber gms
MORNING						
AFTERNOON						
EVENING						
TOTALS						

MY DAILY ACTIVITY

> *"People seldom refuse help, if one offers it in the right way."*
>
> —A. C. BENSON

Someone who has walked a similar path can affect, engage, and inspire in ways that others cannot. How often have we noticed somebody's weight loss and asked them what they're doing to make it happen? If they were willing to share, we usually benefited from their experience, ideas, and suggestions. As people on our own path toward wellness, we also are uniquely qualified to offer others real solutions based on our experience.

We offer help in the right way when we allow our wellness to speak for us, rather than lecturing about it. By allowing people to approach us, rather than approaching them, we eliminate the possibility of inadvertently offending or alienating those who either weren't ready or didn't want or need our solutions.

Today, demonstrate rather than promote your wellness.

Daily Nutritional Information

Time	Amt.	Cal.	Fat gms	Protein gms	Carbs gms	Fiber gms
MORNING						
AFTERNOON						
EVENING						
TOTALS						

MY DAILY ACTIVITY

_____

_____

_____

_____

_____

_____

_____

_____

"Successful people ask better questions, and as a result, they get better answers."

—◦ ANTHONY ROBBINS

*O*ften, the key to having breakthroughs in our fitness efforts is to reframe the questions we ask ourselves. Only negative answers can come from negative questions like "What's the use?" or "How can this help?" If we want positive answers, we need to ask positive questions, such as "How can I?" or "What's the solution?" and maybe even "Why not?"

For example, if we don't see the results we want on the scale after carefully watching the way we eat and ask ourselves "Why should I bother?" we're setting ourselves up to give up on our goals. We can change the question to "How can I accept where I'm at?" or "What other areas of my life have improved?" and find ways to make peace with the pace of our bodies.

Today, pay attention to the questions you ask yourself.

Daily Nutritional Information

Time	Amt.	Cal.	Fat gms	Protein gms	Carbs gms	Fiber gms
MORNING						
AFTERNOON						
EVENING						
TOTALS						

MY DAILY ACTIVITY

*"The impossible we do immediately;
a miracle takes a little longer."*

—◈ SIGN HANGING IN A PHYSICAL THERAPY OFFICE

*I*f our journey to wellness involves physical healing from a bodily condition—whether it's caused by poor eating habits, a disease, or an accident—we can promote healing by following a plan that includes nourishing food, uplifting activities, and positive thoughts.

While taking constructive action, we also need to accept that physical healing takes time. Depending on the circumstances, complete healing can take days, months, even years. In cases where healing isn't going to happen quickly, we get to practice patience and faith along with our physical activities.

Today, accept that healing has its own timetable.

Daily Nutritional Information

Time	Amt.	Cal.	Fat gms	Protein gms	Carbs gms	Fiber gms
MORNING						
AFTERNOON						
EVENING						
TOTALS						

MY DAILY ACTIVITY

> *"We do not stop exercising because we grow old—we grow old because we stop exercising."*
>
> —Dr. Kenneth Cooper

There's no fountain of youth, but exercise can do much the same thing. When we keep moving, we stay flexible and strong in mind and body, generate energy and stamina, and contribute to the health of our bodies' circulatory and immune systems, which in turn helps prevent some age-related diseases.

Because exercise contributes to longevity, we also get to look and feel our best for a longer period of time.

Today, stay young—exercise.

Daily Nutritional Information

Time	Amt.	Cal.	Fat gms	Protein gms	Carbs gms	Fiber gms
MORNING						
AFTERNOON						
EVENING						
TOTALS						

MY DAILY ACTIVITY

"Beginning is easy—continuing hard."

a few months into our fitness efforts, we may start thinking we don't need to work so hard. Maybe we've gotten to a place that feels pretty good and we think we can relax for a while. Or maybe we haven't gotten to the fitness level we hoped for by this time and we're frustrated at what seems like a lot of effort for not enough payoff.

We may need to find some additional motivations to get over the hump and keep going. If we've been doing well, let's congratulate ourselves on our ability to stick to a plan and remind ourselves why we picked the goal we set in the first place. If we're tired and discouraged, we may have to stay positive, recommit to our goal, and perhaps redouble our efforts.

Today, keep going.

Daily Nutritional Information

Time	Amt.	Cal.	Fat gms	Protein gms	Carbs gms	Fiber gms
MORNING						
AFTERNOON						
EVENING						
TOTALS						

My Daily Activity

_____

_____

_____

_____

_____

_____

_____

_____

_____

_____

> "I made a commitment to completely cut out drinking and anything that might hamper me from getting my mind and body together. And the floodgates of goodness have opened upon me—spiritually and financially."
>
> —Ⓢ DENZEL WASHINGTON

The universe is full of infinite blessings. We can have whatever we want in life: health, love, financial abundance, peace of mind, fulfilling work, family. To receive these gifts, we must make ourselves ready by practicing right thinking and right actions.

Right thinking involves choosing positive thoughts, keeping an optimistic attitude, and cultivating a spiritual connection. Right action involves eating well, helping others, and living with integrity. We embrace right living and we open the floodgates of goodness.

Today, commit to right living.

Daily Nutritional Information

Time	Amt.	Cal.	Fat gms	Protein gms	Carbs gms	Fiber gms
MORNING						
AFTERNOON						
EVENING						
TOTALS						

My Daily Activity

_____

_____

_____

_____

_____

_____

_____

_____

_____

_____

"The enlightened give thanks for what most people take for granted . . . As you begin to be grateful for what most people take for granted, the vibration of gratitude makes you more receptive to good in your life."

— THE REV. MICHAEL BECKWITH

*G*ratitude is the gift that keeps on giving. Cultivating gratitude advances our health and self-esteem, and it invites more of what we want into our lives. It acts like a magnet: the more grateful we are for the good things in our lives, the more good things come to us.

As easy as it is to take for granted our everyday blessings, we reap rewards when we take a moment to express gratitude for all we have. Our appreciation for our health, families, friends, or other good things in our lives will enlighten us and attract even more things to appreciate.

Today, have an attitude of gratitude.

Daily Nutritional Information

Time	Amt.	Cal.	Fat gms	Protein gms	Carbs gms	Fiber gms
MORNING						
AFTERNOON						
EVENING						
TOTALS						

MY DAILY ACTIVITY

_____

_____

_____

_____

_____

_____

_____

_____

_____

_____

> *"Our clothes are too much a part of us to ever be entirely indifferent to their condition; it is as though the fabric were indeed a natural extension of the body, or even the soul."*
>
> —QUENTIN BELL

*T*hose of us who've battled with excess weight or poor body image were often so ashamed of our bodies that we wore clothes that didn't fit. We hid under big, baggy, shapeless clothes or we suffered in too-small sizes because we knew we were going to lose weight any day now.

Accepting our bodies as they are, where they are, is part of being fit and well. Acceptance means dressing becomingly. We don't have to spend thousands of dollars on new wardrobes to wear well-fitting attire in patterns, colors, and styles we love. When we dress well, we feel good about ourselves.

Today, wear well-fitting clothes you love.

Daily Nutritional Information

Time	Amt.	Cal.	Fat gms	Protein gms	Carbs gms	Fiber gms
MORNING						
AFTERNOON						
EVENING						
TOTALS						

My Daily Activity

_____

_____

_____

_____

_____

_____

_____

_____

_____

> *"The people who say they don't have time to take care of themselves will soon discover they're spending all their time being sick."*
>
> —◦ PATRICIA ALEXANDER

We may get frustrated at the time we spend taking care of our health. Preparing healthy meals, exercising, and connecting with our friends and loved ones can eat into an already busy schedule.

When we weigh the cost of not taking care of ourselves, however, we can easily see that every minute we spend in self-care is a well-spent investment in our current and future health.

Today, invest time in your health.

Daily Nutritional Information

Time	Amt.	Cal.	Fat gms	Protein gms	Carbs gms	Fiber gms
MORNING						
AFTERNOON						
EVENING						
TOTALS						

MY DAILY ACTIVITY

_____

_____

_____

_____

_____

_____

_____

_____

_____

_____

> "*Every day I walk myself into a state of well-being and walk away from every illness. I have walked myself into my best thoughts, and I know of no thought so burdensome that one cannot walk away from it.*"
>
> —⁊ SØREN KIERKEGAARD

Walking is as good for our minds as it is for our bodies. A good walk gets our heart rates up, clears our heads, calms untamed emotions, and even lulls us into a relaxed meditative state.

We can tailor our walks to our preferences. We can listen to favorite music or none at all. We can walk with a friend or enjoy our solitude. However we do it, we can walk our way to good health, mentally and physically.

Today, walk toward health.

Daily Nutritional Information

Time	Amt.	Cal.	Fat gms	Protein gms	Carbs gms	Fiber gms
MORNING						
AFTERNOON						
EVENING						
TOTALS						

MY DAILY ACTIVITY

_____

_____

_____

_____

_____

_____

_____

_____

_____

_____

> *"For most people, a makeover means losing weight and getting new clothes, hair and makeup. But what they may not know is that the body does its own extreme makeover regularly. In fact, 98 percent of the atoms in the body are replaced yearly."*
>
> —David Kestenbaum

The human body is an amazing, rejuvenating organism. It can reverse years of damage in short periods of time. It can revitalize entire systems. It can fight diseases and send them into remission. Every effort we put forth to properly nourish our bodies, build their strength, and rest them properly aids in our rejuvenation.

It's good to remember, when we wonder whether we can really change our habits and our lives, that our natural state of being is continuous rejuvenation.

Today, forget the hair and makeup—go for the atomic makeover.

Daily Nutritional Information

Time	Amt.	Cal.	Fat gms	Protein gms	Carbs gms	Fiber gms
MORNING						
AFTERNOON						
EVENING						
TOTALS						

MY DAILY ACTIVITY

"Live well. It is the greatest revenge."

—THE TALMUD

D espite the old saying, revenge isn't sweet. It's not sweet when, for instance, seething with rage at somebody or something, we take revenge by "eating at them" in a self-destructive binge. Nor is it sweet when we retaliate with unkind words or actions that leave others hurt and us remorseful. In the end, revenge can be bitter, not sweet.

Fortunately, we can learn to process our anger in healthy ways. Releasing angry energy through exercise, talking to friends, journaling, or meditation lets us work though it without hurting ourselves or others. We then get the benefits of our healthy actions: We look great, we feel great, and we show the world we are mature, gracious, classy people.

Today, savor the sweetness of a life well lived.

Daily Nutritional Information

Time	Amt.	Cal.	Fat gms	Protein gms	Carbs gms	Fiber gms
MORNING						
AFTERNOON						
EVENING						
TOTALS						

MY DAILY ACTIVITY

"I marvel at my own sense of calm now. Events that used to leave me reeling, with my head in a bag of chips, no longer even faze me."

—⟡ OPRAH WINFREY

ortunately, there is hope for those of us who automatically turn to food when the going gets tough. The ability to cope is like a muscle that gets stronger with regular use. Every situation we face without overeating strengthens our coping muscle, increasing our endurance and ability to overcome resistance.

With regular workouts of our coping muscles, we are able to calmly and successfully show up for events, face people, and manage responsibilities that used to leave us reeling. We'll marvel at our own sense of calm.

Today, work your coping muscles.

Daily Nutritional Information

Time	Amt.	Cal.	Fat gms	Protein gms	Carbs gms	Fiber gms
MORNING						
AFTERNOON						
EVENING						
TOTALS						

MY DAILY ACTIVITY

"Intuition is a spiritual faculty and does not explain, but simply points the way."

—⟆ FLORENCE SCOVEL SHINN

Whatever it's called—a gut feeling, a hunch, or a sixth sense—intuition is an inner knowing that just feels right. It's the feeling of "home" when we're in the right place, at the right time, with the right people. It's also the feeling of unrest when we are in the wrong place, at the wrong time, with the wrong people. It's the spiritual faculty that reveals the next steps in our life's journey.

Like a compass discovered in a hidden compartment, our intuition is always with us and will start pointing the way the moment we pay attention to it. The longer we live a life geared toward achieving overall well-being, the stronger our intuition will become, and the more obvious the path we need to take.

Today, practice tuning in to your intuition.

Daily Nutritional Information

Time	Amt.	Cal.	Fat gms	Protein gms	Carbs gms	Fiber gms
MORNING						
AFTERNOON						
EVENING						
TOTALS						

My Daily Activity

_____

_____

_____

_____

_____

_____

_____

_____

_____

"The first problem for all of us, men and women, is not to learn, but to unlearn."

— GLORIA STEINEM

To learn entails not just acquiring new knowledge; we also have to unlearn what no longer serves us. This doesn't mean we have to toss out all our accumulated experiences or presume everything we know is wrong. Rather, unlearning simply requires we become open to new and different skills, experiences, and behaviors.

Unlearning is a process. For example, we can unlearn stuffing feelings down with food when we're upset and instead learn to communicate effectively. We can unlearn rushing through meals and learn to eat slowly and really taste our food. As we progress, we can place our old knowledge in a mental storage box, attach a sign that says, "Things That No Longer Serve Me," and move forward.

Today, unlearn at least one thing.

Daily Nutritional Information

Time	Amt.	Cal.	Fat gms	Protein gms	Carbs gms	Fiber gms
MORNING						
AFTERNOON						
EVENING						
TOTALS						

My Daily Activity

> *"The most important single aspect of software development is to be clear about what you are trying to build."*
>
> —⌕ BJARNE STROUSTRUP

Like a computer, a belief system doesn't judge the data we input; it simply accepts it as fact. Therefore, our belief systems accept both positive and negative feedback equally—beliefs of confidence and success can be developed just as effectively as beliefs of inadequacy and limitation.

As our own computer programmers, we get to decide what programs we want to run. We get to delete old negative beliefs input by previous users and reprogram affirmations of health, well-being, and happiness. We can delete old habits that don't work and upload new ones that do. By carefully selecting the data, we can program our lives exactly to our own spectacular specifications.

Today, input only positive data.

Daily Nutritional Information

Time	Amt.	Cal.	Fat gms	Protein gms	Carbs gms	Fiber gms
MORNING						
AFTERNOON						
EVENING						
TOTALS						

My Daily Activity

"Any emotion, if it is sincere, is involuntary."

—Ꙩ MARK TWAIN

People are creatures of emotion—and not everybody is happy about this. For those of us with tendencies to turn to food when uncomfortable feelings arise, emotions can be just as unwelcome as uninvited visitors— we're displeased when they knock on the door and we have no idea what to do with them once they're here.

There is hope for the emotion averse. We can make peace with our feelings by accepting them as natural and healthy parts of our makeup. This allows us to put our energy into learning to process our feelings in positive ways rather than trying to fight them.

Today, recognize your emotions as healthy.

Daily Nutritional Information

Time	Amt.	Cal.	Fat gms	Protein gms	Carbs gms	Fiber gms
MORNING						
AFTERNOON						
EVENING						
TOTALS						

MY DAILY ACTIVITY

_____

_____

_____

_____

_____

_____

_____

_____

_____

"When I get a new idea, I start at once building it up in my imagination . . . when I see no fault anywhere, I put into concrete form the final product of my brain."

—Nikola Tesla

Like any invention, the first step to creating the healthy, dynamic life we want is to visualize it. First, we need to form and refine in our minds exactly what we want, whether it's to achieve optimal health, lose excess weight, or increase muscular strength. Our clarity will enable us to take inspired, focused action to achieve our goals.

Today, focus first; act second.

Daily Nutritional Information

Time	Amt.	Cal.	Fat gms	Protein gms	Carbs gms	Fiber gms
MORNING						
AFTERNOON						
EVENING						
TOTALS						

MY DAILY ACTIVITY

_____

_____

_____

_____

_____

_____

_____

_____

_____

"Relinquish your attachment to the known, step into the unknown, and you will step into the field of all possibilities."

—⟩ DEEPAK CHOPRA

We may think about wellness in terms of relatively small goals: changing a food plan, starting an exercise program, getting to bed earlier. Having goals is important to our success, but overall wellness is much bigger. It's really relinquishing one way of life and stepping into another.

We may be anxious about changing. What will life be like if we give up certain foods and get exercise every day? How will we feel, physically, mentally, and emotionally? Who will we be? The road to wellness may take us places we can't even imagine right now.

Today, view change as a step into new possibilities.

Daily Nutritional Information

Time	Amt.	Cal.	Fat gms	Protein gms	Carbs gms	Fiber gms
MORNING						
AFTERNOON						
EVENING						
TOTALS						

MY DAILY ACTIVITY

"When it comes to eating right and exercising, there is no 'I'll start tomorrow.' Tomorrow is a disease."

—V. L. Allineare

How tempting it is to put off until tomorrow what we could do today. We're just too busy today to eat right or exercise or get enough sleep. Maybe we're too tired, or too emotionally fragile, or just feeling overwhelmed. We'll take today off and start again tomorrow.

When we start putting off positive action until "tomorrow," we risk never starting at all. If we find that we just cannot get moving, a buddy system may be the perfect solution. Other people can give us the encouragement and accountability we need to get started. If we tell a supportive friend our intentions, we're more likely to follow through. Once we start, we'll develop momentum that will help us get going and keep going—starting today.

Today, beat procrastination with a little help from your friends.

Daily Nutritional Information

Time	Amt.	Cal.	Fat gms	Protein gms	Carbs gms	Fiber gms
MORNING						
AFTERNOON						
EVENING						
TOTALS						

MY DAILY ACTIVITY

_____

_____

_____

_____

_____

_____

_____

_____

_____

> *"Every human being is the author of his own health or disease."*
>
> —☙ BUDDHA

When it comes to our health, we can choose from a variety of approaches, everything from traditional and alternative medicines to folk remedies to spiritual and religious practices. Whether we work with a practitioner or not, ultimately our health is our responsibility—nobody knows our one and only bodies better than we do.

We get our best results when we view practitioners as partners in our well-being. It is our responsibility to clearly communicate our needs and preferences and our aches and pains so they can prescribe treatment that is right for us. Once we are certain we are working with the right practitioner and have the right treatment, we can take direction with confidence, knowing our best interests are being served.

Today, be an active participant in your own health.

Daily Nutritional Information

Time	Amt.	Cal.	Fat gms	Protein gms	Carbs gms	Fiber gms
MORNING						
AFTERNOON						
EVENING						
TOTALS						

MY DAILY ACTIVITY

_____

_____

_____

_____

_____

_____

_____

_____

_____

> *"The only person who likes change is a wet baby."*
>
> —⌇ ROY BLITZER

Change is a word that strikes terror into the hearts of millions. We know we need to improve our eating habits. We know we need to get up and get moving. We know we need to let go of certain foods, behaviors, and habits. We even know we'll feel better when we do. But we're not happy about it. Fortunately, we don't have to like change—we just have to make it.

Luckily, we don't have to change everything at once to gain lasting benefits. We can improve our lives and reach our goals by taking small, steady, and consistent steps. Taking it one change at a time allows us to adjust, get comfortable, and gear up for the next change. We may never like change, but we can come to view it as an opportunity for growth and appreciate the benefits it brings.

Today, take it one change at a time.

Daily Nutritional Information

Time	Amt.	Cal.	Fat gms	Protein gms	Carbs gms	Fiber gms
MORNING						
AFTERNOON						
EVENING						
TOTALS						

MY DAILY ACTIVITY

> "We need quiet time to examine our lives openly and honestly—spending quiet time alone gives your mind an opportunity to renew itself and create order."
>
> —⌒ SUSAN TAYLOR

*J*ust like healthy food and exercise, quiet time is an essential ingredient in a complete wellness program. How much time do we give ourselves to really think about our lives? When we don't give ourselves the luxury of quiet time, we lose the opportunity to obtain emotional and spiritual renewal.

It's important to spend time each week, month, or year to reflect on where we've been, are now, and want to go. Living in the accelerated modern world can make it especially tough to carve out quality quiet time. But, even if our schedules allow only the occasional stolen hour, we can greatly benefit from the insight that comes with solitude. No phone calls. No e-mails. No interruptions, except from the thoughts we capture inside the quiet.

Today, steal some quiet time.

Daily Nutritional Information

Time	Amt.	Cal.	Fat gms	Protein gms	Carbs gms	Fiber gms
MORNING						
AFTERNOON						
EVENING						
TOTALS						

MY DAILY ACTIVITY

"Making mistakes, getting it almost right, and experimenting to see what happens are all part of the process of eventually getting it right."

—JACK CANFIELD

If we're having a hard time staying on track, it's important we stay positive no matter how many attempts we make. Each new effort takes us closer to the one that will work. Eventually we will get it right.

Getting and staying fit isn't a matter of taking an action and getting a specific result. We're all different, our bodies are all different. We have to use a process of trial and error to figure out what will work best for us as we work toward a healthy life.

Today, do not give up.

Daily Nutritional Information

Time	Amt.	Cal.	Fat gms	Protein gms	Carbs gms	Fiber gms
MORNING						
AFTERNOON						
EVENING						
TOTALS						

My Daily Activity

_____

_____

_____

_____

_____

_____

_____

_____

_____

_____

"Sometimes the most important thing in a whole day is the rest we take between two deep breaths."

—Etty Hillesum

One of the healthiest, most effective, and more powerful stress-relieving tools is available to us right here, right now, and it's free, easy, and requires no equipment: two breaths. Taking two deep breaths when we're frazzled or unsettled is all most of us need to center our minds, collect our thoughts, and find peace.

Eyes closed or open, deeply inhaling, holding our breath for a moment, exhaling and then repeating gives us the pause we need to connect to the stillness within. When we return to our activities, we are clear, centered, and connected.

Today, take two deep breaths and rest your mind.

Daily Nutritional Information

Time	Amt.	Cal.	Fat gms	Protein gms	Carbs gms	Fiber gms
MORNING						
AFTERNOON						
EVENING						
TOTALS						

MY DAILY ACTIVITY

_____

_____

_____

_____

_____

_____

_____

_____

_____

Month 5

Celebrate Progress

> "The first step in becoming a Spiritual Master is to love your body as much as God loves the earth and to give up the idea of killing it."
>
> —⨀ SONDRA RAY

*E*very bite of nourishing food we take is a choice to live, to love our bodies, and to leave our old habits behind. Every set of exercises we do, every walk we take, every stretch, is a choice to help our bodies be healthy and strong.

The inescapable physical and spiritual connection means that the more lovingly we treat our bodies, the more lovingly we feel toward them, and the more we grow spiritually.

Today, love your body.

Daily Nutritional Information

Time	Amt.	Cal.	Fat gms	Protein gms	Carbs gms	Fiber gms
MORNING						
AFTERNOON						
EVENING						
TOTALS						

MY DAILY ACTIVITY

"The difference between a reaction and a response is three breaths."

—Ⓢ Anonymous

For many of us, eating when we're upset or stressed is such an automatic reaction that we've often found ourselves with food in our mouths before we even realize it. Learning to recognize when we're impulsively reacting to a situation allows us to have thoughtful, controlled responses instead.

Taking three deep breaths forces us to pause and consider our options before that first compulsive bite. Can we step away from the frustrating task at hand? Can we call someone for help? In the time we pause, we can find an appropriate response to whatever is going on, rather than an unthinking reaction.

Today, don't react—respond.

Daily Nutritional Information

Time	Amt.	Cal.	Fat gms	Protein gms	Carbs gms	Fiber gms
MORNING						
AFTERNOON						
EVENING						
TOTALS						

My Daily Activity

> *"Do not look where you fell, but where you slipped."*
>
> —AFRICAN PROVERB

M istakes, missteps, mishaps—we've all done them. Whether it is unintentionally insulting somebody at a party, forgetting a birthday, or deviating from our food and exercise plans, slipping up in life is not a catastrophe but an opportunity for learning and changing.

Evaluating what led to the slip gives us valuable information to make better choices in the future. The only real mistake is to miss the valuable lessons every slip can teach.

Today, learn from your mistakes.

Daily Nutritional Information

Time	Amt.	Cal.	Fat gms	Protein gms	Carbs gms	Fiber gms
MORNING						
AFTERNOON						
EVENING						
TOTALS						

MY DAILY ACTIVITY

"And, finally, the most important breakup rule. No matter who broke your heart or how long it takes to heal, you'll never get through it without your friends."

— CARRIE BRADSHAW (SARAH JESSICA PARKER)
IN *SEX AND THE CITY*

Whether we need a shoulder to cry on or someone to celebrate with, life is best shared over friendship. Just as our houses and bodies don't maintain themselves, friendships have to be kept up and nurtured. No matter how busy we are, few things are better investments of our time than friendships.

Maintaining friendships can be as simple as sending out regular e-mails to friends we don't often see or as involved as setting up regularly scheduled dinners. Every effort counts and helps build the long-lasting, loving friendships that enrich our lives.

Today, do one thing to nurture a friendship.

Daily Nutritional Information

Time	Amt.	Cal.	Fat gms	Protein gms	Carbs gms	Fiber gms
MORNING						
AFTERNOON						
EVENING						
TOTALS						

MY DAILY ACTIVITY

"One may go a long way after one is tired."

We're challenging ourselves with healthy physical activity and we're feeling it—our arms ache, our legs are tired, and our abs are crying "uncle." At times like these, it can be tempting to stop before we've gotten our full health benefits. It's time to kick our mental strategies into high gear; it's time for mind over muscle.

A few simple mental techniques can keep us going. Repeating positive, encouraging statements; reminding ourselves we only have a little longer to go; or visualizing ourselves achieving our goals helps us stay tough, focused—and moving.

Today, train your brain and your body.

Daily Nutritional Information

Time	Amt.	Cal.	Fat gms	Protein gms	Carbs gms	Fiber gms
MORNING						
AFTERNOON						
EVENING						
TOTALS						

My Daily Activity

_____

_____

_____

_____

_____

_____

_____

_____

_____

_____

"Energy is eternal delight."

—WILLIAM BLAKE

We can buy almost anything in today's world—including energy. We can find products with artificial stimulants online and in most grocery, convenience, and drug stores. We may get the immediate blast of feel-good energy that comes in a bottle, can, cup, or pill, but if we're dependent on or overuse chemicals to meet our basic daily functions, we'll ultimately be left even more exhausted on deeper levels.

Real energy comes from real wellness—proper nutrition, rest, and emotional and spiritual balance. Living well unleashes reserves of energy that boost our immune systems and allow us to meet our challenges with more vigor and stamina than we could ever buy.

Today, tap into your natural energy reserves.

Daily Nutritional Information

Time	Amt.	Cal.	Fat gms	Protein gms	Carbs gms	Fiber gms
MORNING						
AFTERNOON						
EVENING						
TOTALS						

MY DAILY ACTIVITY

> "When you carry out acts of kindness, you get a wonderful feeling inside. It is as though something inside your body responds and says, yes, this is how I ought to feel."
>
> —⟋ HAROLD KUSHNER

We know the kind acts we do have a profound impact on others, but we may not realize the positive impact they also have on ourselves. With every kind act we perform, we increase our self-worth, happiness, and optimism.

The ripples of kindness can extend far beyond our immediate reach. When we offer a kindness, such as opening a door for a stranger or giving a stranded friend a ride, we demonstrate to others what kindness looks like. They may then be inspired to perform their own acts of kindness, which can inspire others, who inspire yet others . . . We shouldn't underestimate the impact a kind act can have on the world.

Today, do one random act of kindness.

Daily Nutritional Information

Time	Amt.	Cal.	Fat gms	Protein gms	Carbs gms	Fiber gms
MORNING						
AFTERNOON						
EVENING						
TOTALS						

My Daily Activity

_____

_____

_____

_____

_____

_____

_____

_____

_____

> *"There is no success but your own success."*
>
> —ᯤ LESLIE GRIMUTTER

*a*s we become healthier and see our bodies changing, it's important we acknowledge all our successes, not just the ones that can be measured on the scale, in inches, or in test results.

Did we meet a challenge with new confidence? Have we made a surprising discovery about our abilities, talents, or potential? Was it hard for us to say no to something not good for us—but we did it anyway? Recognizing our successes makes us feel good and is the surest way to have more success in the future.

Today, acknowledge your successes.

Daily Nutritional Information

Time	Amt.	Cal.	Fat gms	Protein gms	Carbs gms	Fiber gms
MORNING						
AFTERNOON						
EVENING						
TOTALS						

MY DAILY ACTIVITY

_____

_____

_____

_____

_____

_____

_____

_____

_____

"A vacation is what you take when you can no longer take what you've been taking."

—Ꙅ EARL WILSON

Rejuvenation is an important part of wellness—and that means taking vacations. We don't have to take weeklong cruises or trips abroad to refresh ourselves. We have an array of vacation choices available to fit our needs, schedules, and budgets.

Organized retreats, weekend getaways, even a week spent at home without stress can allow us to rest, break up the monotony of our daily routines, and enable us to regroup and recharge.

Today, plan some vacation therapy.

Daily Nutritional Information

Time	Amt.	Cal.	Fat gms	Protein gms	Carbs gms	Fiber gms
MORNING						
AFTERNOON						
EVENING						
TOTALS						

MY DAILY ACTIVITY

> "Motivation is a fire from within. If someone else tries to light that fire under you, chances are it will burn very briefly."
>
> —Stephen R. Covey

Embracing a healthy lifestyle is like any other long-term change—we need to be properly motivated or eventually we'll stop working at it. Our motivations are as varied as we are.

Some of us are seeking wellness because we were given a diagnosis that requires we take care of our bodies in a new way. Others are walking the road of recovery from compulsive eating, undereating, or bingeing and purging. Still others do it because there are pounds to lose, muscles to strengthen, countries to visit, and grandkids to spoil. Whatever our reasons, they must be meaningful, personal, and strong enough to sustain us for the long haul.

Today, discover your motivations for seeking wellness.

Daily Nutritional Information

Time	Amt.	Cal.	Fat gms	Protein gms	Carbs gms	Fiber gms
MORNING						
AFTERNOON						
EVENING						
TOTALS						

MY DAILY ACTIVITY

> *"People often say that motivation doesn't last. Well, neither does bathing—that's why we recommend it daily."*
>
> —ZIG ZIGLAR

We remember the day we decided to embark on the path toward a healthy lifestyle. Maybe it was because we couldn't get a favorite pair of pants zipped, or because we realized that we were completely out of breath after climbing just one set of stairs, or because our doctor told us that we had to. Whatever the motivation, we knew we had to make real change and we committed to it.

Once we see progress—pants may zip more easily and a set of stairs no longer fazes us—it's easy to lose track of our initial motivation. We may need to remind ourselves why we started this journey and then recommit to our goals. It's important to acknowledge and celebrate the progress we've made—and equally important to keep going.

Today, remind yourself of the reasons you decided to seek a healthy lifestyle.

Daily Nutritional Information

Time	Amt.	Cal.	Fat gms	Protein gms	Carbs gms	Fiber gms
MORNING						
AFTERNOON						
EVENING						
TOTALS						

MY DAILY ACTIVITY

> "I fall back on this Journal just as some other poor devil takes to drink."
>
> —W. N. P. BARBELLION

To keep our commitment to wellness, we may need to find a healthy outlet for our feelings. For many, journal writing is the perfect solution. Journals allow us to "binge on paper"—to purge our feelings by writing them down instead of stuffing them with food.

Journals are private, inexpensive, and travel well. Words flow freely for some; others struggle to pick up what often feels like the hundred-pound pen. In either case, though, insight, clarity, and healing are always available through the written journey.

Today, write in a journal.

Daily Nutritional Information

Time	Amt.	Cal.	Fat gms	Protein gms	Carbs gms	Fiber gms
MORNING						
AFTERNOON						
EVENING						
TOTALS						

My Daily Activity

"It is better to take many small steps in the right direction than to make a great leap forward only to stumble backward."

—⟩ CHINESE PROVERB

*I*f we find we're having a hard time staying on track—or getting back after a lapse—the problem may not be lack of motivation, it may be fear. The idea of really changing our lives can be daunting, enough to paralyze us.

Rather than stress ourselves trying to change everything at once, we need to remind ourselves that getting and staying healthy is a lifetime journey, not an overnight adventure. We don't need to change our lives at once, just to make the healthy changes we can, today.

Today, take just one step toward health.

Daily Nutritional Information

Time	Amt.	Cal.	Fat gms	Protein gms	Carbs gms	Fiber gms
MORNING						
AFTERNOON						
EVENING						
TOTALS						

My Daily Activity

_____

_____

_____

_____

_____

_____

_____

_____

_____

"The key is not to prioritize what's on your schedule, but to schedule your priorities."

—Stephen R. Covey

Demands on our time can cause us to make poor choices that compromise our health: We hit the drive-through instead of the grocery store, do our paperwork instead of a workout, and eat in front of the refrigerator instead of at the table. When life is in full session, we need to step back and ask ourselves: What's my priority?

Keeping health a priority means putting it on our schedules—literally. Putting self-care activities like grocery shopping, workouts, and doctor appointments on our calendars allows us to build schedules around our health.

Today, put self-care activities on your schedule.

Daily Nutritional Information

Time	Amt.	Cal.	Fat gms	Protein gms	Carbs gms	Fiber gms
MORNING						
AFTERNOON						
EVENING						
TOTALS						

MY DAILY ACTIVITY

> "Getting out of shape is like a thief in the night that sneaks up on you. I always tell people that it is never too late. I tell them about the folks in their nineties that doubled their strength and endurance."
>
> —JACK LALANNE

*I*t's never too late to start taking care of our health. No matter how far down (or up) the scale we have gone, there is always positive action we can take to cultivate wellness. Our bodies are remarkable in their abilities to recover, heal, and gain new strength and stamina. As long as there is breath in our bodies, we can improve.

Sometimes we think there's no point in trying to get healthier: We're too old, we're too tired, we've been doing things in an unhealthy way for too long. We can get rid of those excuses and remind ourselves that healthy living will make us feel better, no matter how old we are.

Today, remember that it's not too late to get healthy.

Daily Nutritional Information

Time	Amt.	Cal.	Fat gms	Protein gms	Carbs gms	Fiber gms
MORNING						
AFTERNOON						
EVENING						
TOTALS						

My Daily Activity

_____

_____

_____

_____

_____

_____

_____

_____

_____

"I've learned that you shouldn't go through life with a catcher's mitt on both hands. You need to be able to throw something back."

—⌒ MAYA ANGELOU

*J*ust as in the game of baseball, successful living involves teamwork. Being a member of a team means carrying our own weight. During our trying times, we should freely take the support, encouragement, and guidance our teammates offer. Their help allows us to heal from our injuries, rebuild our muscles, and regain our focus.

Once back in the game, it's time for us to be there for our teammates when they need us. A solid give-and-take strategy is the secret to a winning game.

Today, throw as much as you catch.

Daily Nutritional Information

Time	Amt.	Cal.	Fat gms	Protein gms	Carbs gms	Fiber gms
MORNING						
AFTERNOON						
EVENING						
TOTALS						

MY DAILY ACTIVITY

"The willingness to accept responsibility for one's own life is the source from which self-respect springs."

—JOAN DIDION

Being responsible for ourselves involves more than just taking care of our bodies. We also need to take charge of our long-term care. Setting up healthcare plans, financial budgets, insurance policies, and retirement accounts helps ensure that we and our loved ones get proper care.

The paperwork for these health essentials can be intimidating—enough so that we're tempted to put off dealing with it, or to ignore it altogether. Some of us don't like to think about getting ill or even dying, so we avoid getting the protection everyone needs. But when we put these resources in place, we put our care into the right hands: our own.

Today, be responsible for your own well-being.

Daily Nutritional Information

Time	Amt.	Cal.	Fat gms	Protein gms	Carbs gms	Fiber gms
MORNING						
AFTERNOON						
EVENING						
TOTALS						

My Daily Activity

> *"Don't let your mouth write no check that your tail can't cash."*
>
> —Bo Diddley

Sometimes our mouths have minds of their own. How many times have we heard them say yes to yet another commitment when our heads knew we should say no? When we overextend our time, energy, and resources, we risk not being able to fulfill our commitments, which can strain our relationships and erode our self-esteem. Saying yes to too many activities often results in overcrowded schedules, exhausted bodies, and, often, overeating.

As difficult as it can be, we need to say no. This simple two-letter word empowers us to take charge of our schedules—and our sanity.

Today, learn to say no.

Daily Nutritional Information

Time	Amt.	Cal.	Fat gms	Protein gms	Carbs gms	Fiber gms
MORNING						
AFTERNOON						
EVENING						
TOTALS						

My Daily Activity

_____

_____

_____

_____

_____

_____

_____

_____

_____

> *"Few things are harder to put up with than a good example."*
>
> — MARK TWAIN

Who hasn't compared his body to another's fit physique and found himself falling short? Envy can actually be a helpful tool if we use it as an inspiration for greater things. When it spurs self-destructive and self-defeating thoughts, however, envy can roadblock our success.

The key is to use those we admire as examples. If we see someone with the toned arms we want, for example, perhaps we can incorporate more strength training into our routines. Maybe we meet a yoga devotee whose serenity inspires us to try a class. When we turn envy to admiration, we can use it to achieve higher goals.

Today, turn envy into incentive.

Daily Nutritional Information

Time	Amt.	Cal.	Fat gms	Protein gms	Carbs gms	Fiber gms
MORNING						
AFTERNOON						
EVENING						
TOTALS						

MY DAILY ACTIVITY

> "I have accepted fear as a part of life—
> specifically the fear of change. . . . I
> have gone ahead despite the pounding in
> the heart that says: turn back."
>
> —ERICA JONG

It's easy to notice positive changes in our minds and bodies and then panic. What will life look like if I am fit and healthy? What if I get attention from the opposite sex? We need to make sure we don't sabotage ourselves as we create healthier lives.

Fear of change is the root cause of self-sabotage. When we see change and start to panic, we need to take deep breaths and turn to our support systems for help. Tapping into the experience of other people who have changed their lives successfully can be the key to soothing our nerves and reassuring us that change is healthy, good—and survivable.

Today, watch for self-sabotaging behaviors.

Daily Nutritional Information

Time	Amt.	Cal.	Fat gms	Protein gms	Carbs gms	Fiber gms
MORNING						
AFTERNOON						
EVENING						
TOTALS						

My Daily Activity

_____

_____

_____

_____

_____

_____

_____

_____

_____

> *"Whatever you think you can do or believe you can do, begin it. Action has magic, grace, and power in it."*
>
> —JOHANN WOLFGANG VON GOETHE

Wouldn't it be nice if there were a magic wand that, when waved, brought us healthy, fulfilling lives and helped us realize our full potential? There's no magic wand, but there is a magic word: action.

When we think about taking action, we may think only of drastic action, but that's usually not necessary. In fact, making extreme changes can undermine our long-term goals; we may overwhelm ourselves with change we're not ready for. The best kind of action is balanced, consistent, and positive. We can create our best lives, one healthy action at a time.

Today, get into healthy action.

Daily Nutritional Information

Time	Amt.	Cal.	Fat gms	Protein gms	Carbs gms	Fiber gms
MORNING						
AFTERNOON						
EVENING						
TOTALS						

MY DAILY ACTIVITY

_____

_____

_____

_____

_____

_____

_____

_____

_____

"No man in the world has more courage than the man who can stop after eating one peanut."

—CHANNING POLLOCK

Our plates are loaded with fresh, nourishing food, yet our weight's not moving down the scale—what could be the problem? It could be portion sizes. Even if we are eating only healthy food, if we're eating too much, we're still overeating.

Some of us weigh and measure our food as part of a daily routine; others just check occasionally to make sure our portions are right. Some of us memorize the image of appropriate portions and carry that with us. However we do it, regularly checking on the size of the portions we take can keep us from supersizing our portions and halting our progress.

Today, check your portion sizes.

Daily Nutritional Information

Time	Amt.	Cal.	Fat gms	Protein gms	Carbs gms	Fiber gms
MORNING						
AFTERNOON						
EVENING						
TOTALS						

MY DAILY ACTIVITY

"Our bodies communicate to us clearly and specifically, if we are willing to listen to them."

—⧼ SHAKTI GAWAIN

*O*ur wellness programs require we work with and not against our bodies, which means listening to their signals. We can hear what they're saying when we take a quiet moment to close our eyes, breathe, and pay attention to how our bodies are feeling.

If we stopped worrying about how many calories we just ate, and trying to determine if we ate the right protein/carb ratio, or berating ourselves for eating the whole thing, we might learn a lot from our bodies. Perhaps we'll discover that our bodies feel warm and comfortable after a meal, or we'll learn that a food we always believed was healthy for us doesn't feel good in our stomachs. The information is there—we just need to hear it.

Today, practice listening to your body.

Daily Nutritional Information

Time	Amt.	Cal.	Fat gms	Protein gms	Carbs gms	Fiber gms
MORNING						
AFTERNOON						
EVENING						
TOTALS						

MY DAILY ACTIVITY

_____

_____

_____

_____

_____

_____

_____

_____

_____

_____

> *"When you recover or discover something that nourishes your soul and brings joy, care enough about yourself to make room for it in your life."*
>
> —JEAN SHINODA BOLEN

We need to nourish our spiritual selves just as we do our physical selves. Spirituality gives us strength, insight, and inner peace. It's important to make time to develop our spirituality because losing our connection to a greater purpose can leave us feeling lost, purposeless, and disconnected.

The sources for spiritual sustenance are plentiful and varied. Some of us go to a formal place of worship; others find fulfillment in nature, yoga, or community service. We can take whatever path we choose, as long as it leads to calm, comfort, and connection.

Today, make time to nourish your spiritual self.

Daily Nutritional Information

Time	Amt.	Cal.	Fat gms	Protein gms	Carbs gms	Fiber gms
MORNING						
AFTERNOON						
EVENING						
TOTALS						

MY DAILY ACTIVITY

_____

_____

_____

_____

_____

_____

_____

_____

_____

> *"Visualize this thing that you want. See it, feel it, believe in it. Make your mental blueprint, and begin to build!"*
>
> — ROBERT COLLIER

The brain is a highly efficient system that is divided into left and right sides. The left is the side in charge of memory, logic, and rational thought. The right side is responsible for imagination, creativity, and intuition. It holds images, which are the language through which the mind and body communicate.

When we visualize, we are using the right side of our brain. This is why visualization is so powerful in accomplishing our goals; it gives us an automatic mind–body connection.

Today, visualize what you'd like your life to be.

Daily Nutritional Information

Time	Amt.	Cal.	Fat gms	Protein gms	Carbs gms	Fiber gms
MORNING						
AFTERNOON						
EVENING						
TOTALS						

MY DAILY ACTIVITY

"You must see your goals clearly and specifically before you can set out for them. Hold them in your mind until they become second nature."

—⌒ LES BROWN

a healthy lifestyle is made of daily—or even hourly—decisions to choose what is right for our bodies, but it's also created through long-term goals about how we want to live. A decision to avoid unhealthy snacks, or to do an exercise routine today, makes sense as part of a plan to attain or stay at a healthy weight and to increase our overall fitness.

We should have a picture in our heads about what we want our healthier life to be. We also need to map out the specific goals we want to accomplish on our way to that healthier life. Do we want to lose a certain number of pounds? To have a lower resting heart rate? To be able to run a 10K—or a marathon? If we are clear about the goals, we are more likely to make our vision of a healthy life a reality.

Today, write down three goals you'd like to achieve this year.

Daily Nutritional Information

Time	Amt.	Cal.	Fat gms	Protein gms	Carbs gms	Fiber gms
MORNING						
AFTERNOON						
EVENING						
TOTALS						

MY DAILY ACTIVITY

> "We are only as sick as our secrets."
>
> — Anonymous

Most of us have secrets that make us feel ashamed and embarrassed. We think that if anyone knew about our past or some things we said or did, they would reject us or think we were bad. Our secrets isolate us psychologically and cause stress, which set us up for emotional and physical illness.

Peace of mind and health are the gifts we receive when we break our isolation and trust our secrets to a loving person. Turning to a close friend, family member, minister, or therapist, we can evoke healing and a sense of community when we clean our conscience.

Today, trust someone with a secret.

Daily Nutritional Information

Time	Amt.	Cal.	Fat gms	Protein gms	Carbs gms	Fiber gms
MORNING						
AFTERNOON						
EVENING						
TOTALS						

MY DAILY ACTIVITY

> *"There's a lot of people in this world who spend so much time watching their health that they haven't the time to enjoy it."*
>
> —Josh Billings

We woke up early this morning and got in an hour of exercise. Then we sat down to a healthy, low-calorie, high-fiber, high-antioxidants breakfast. We took a multivitamin. Maybe we even got in a few minutes of deep breathing and meditation. In short, we were very good at working toward wellness.

Are we having fun yet? We may want to have a healthy lifestyle so we will live longer or so that we're able to do more. But if all of our efforts are aimed at getting to wellness, rather than enjoying the journey, we need to stop for a moment. The healthy breakfast, exercise, breathing, etc., should help us feel good, not just virtuous.

Today, enjoy your health.

Daily Nutritional Information

Time	Amt.	Cal.	Fat gms	Protein gms	Carbs gms	Fiber gms
MORNING						
AFTERNOON						
EVENING						
TOTALS						

My Daily Activity

> *"The most essential factor is persistence—the determination never to allow your energy or enthusiasm to be dampened by the discouragement that must inevitably come."*
>
> —JAMES WHITCOMB RILEY

*a*t some point, we're likely to get discouraged about developing a healthy lifestyle. If we're trying to lose weight, we may hit a plateau, where the pounds just aren't coming off. If we're working on an exercise program, we may find we can't add any extra weights, or that we're just not able to run as far or as fast as we hoped by this time.

It's important to understand that plateaus in weight loss and fitness are normal. The difference between those who succeed for the long term and those who don't isn't courage or intelligence or even metabolism; it's simply persistence.

Today, persist in your wellness.

Daily Nutritional Information

Time	Amt.	Cal.	Fat gms	Protein gms	Carbs gms	Fiber gms
MORNING						
AFTERNOON						
EVENING						
TOTALS						

MY DAILY ACTIVITY

_____

_____

_____

_____

_____

_____

_____

_____

_____

"If you're tired and pooped out all the time, do you have love and compassion in your heart for your fellow man? You don't even like yourself!"

—JACK LALANNE

ealthy food and appropriate exercise tend to make us have more energy, but there's a third element that's essential—and that we too often neglect: sleep. Too many of us go to bed late and get up early, skimping on sleep we need. Whether it's six hours or ten, our bodies will tell us how much sleep we need to function at our best, if we let them.

Without enough sleep, we are less alert, more irritable, less productive, and more likely to have accidents. When we are sleep-deprived, our immune system can be weakened, making it more likely that we'll get sick or that we'll have a harder time recovering from any injury.

Today, get some sleep.

Daily Nutritional Information

Time	Amt.	Cal.	Fat gms	Protein gms	Carbs gms	Fiber gms
MORNING						
AFTERNOON						
EVENING						
TOTALS						

MY DAILY ACTIVITY

_____

_____

_____

_____

_____

_____

_____

_____

_____

"Food has replaced sex in my life; now, I can't even get into my own pants."

—Anonymous

Whether we are gay or straight, old or young, married or single, sexuality is a healthy, natural, and meaningful part of our makeup. If we've replaced sex with food, it's time to separate the two.

Our sexual attitudes are as diverse as we are. Some of us have hidden or downplayed our sexuality as a result of bad experiences. Others have had too many negative body issues to comfortably explore sexual relationships. Still others have always had healthy sexual viewpoints, which are enhanced by seeking wellness. Whatever our circumstances, and wherever we are in our path toward wellness, we can adopt healthy, positive views of our sexuality.

Today, separate your kitchen from your bedroom.

Daily Nutritional Information

Time	Amt.	Cal.	Fat gms	Protein gms	Carbs gms	Fiber gms
MORNING						
AFTERNOON						
EVENING						
TOTALS						

MY DAILY ACTIVITY

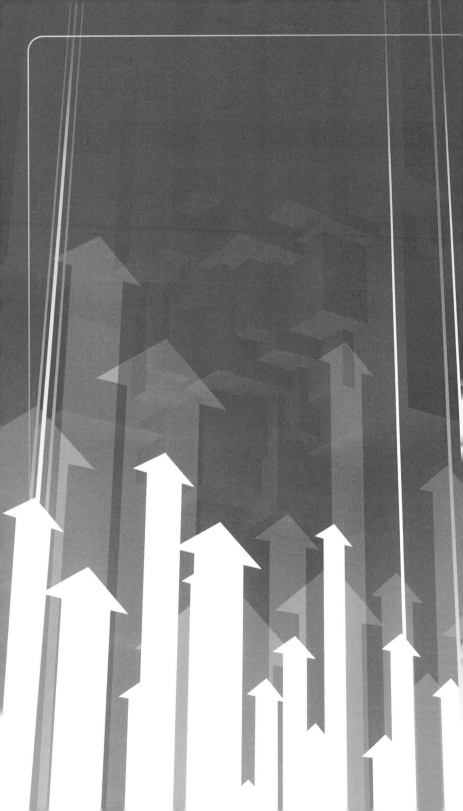

Month 6

Keep Going

> *"I know too well the poison and the sting of things too sweet."*
>
> —☙ ADELAIDE PROCTOR

Who among us hasn't given in to temptation and impulsively eaten food we know isn't good for us? As good as unhealthy food makes us feel in the moment, it makes us feel worse in the long run. The next time we crave something unhealthy, we need to ask ourselves "Is this good for me?" as opposed to "Does this make me feel good right now?"

Pausing and evaluating the long-term consequences of poor choices allows our rational self to override our impulses. Every time we say no to unhealthy food, we say yes to long-term health and happiness.

Today, make only choices that are good for you.

Daily Nutritional Information

Time	Amt.	Cal.	Fat gms	Protein gms	Carbs gms	Fiber gms
MORNING						
AFTERNOON						
EVENING						
TOTALS						

MY DAILY ACTIVITY

_____

_____

_____

_____

_____

_____

_____

_____

_____

> *"The ability to deal with a crisis by putting it within the context of your whole life is part of holistic healing."*
>
> —Ⓢ ROBERT L. KINAST

Some of us live with chronic conditions or diagnoses that dominate our awareness. Since our health issues demand much of our time and attention, it's easy to start to identify ourselves in terms of the condition and miss our overall beauty.

In truth, our conditions are only part of our whole beings. We can choose language that moves the condition from the center of our identity to being simply one part of our whole. Instead of identifying as "a depressive," for example, we can identify as a person with bouts of depression. We can address and acknowledge our conditions, but not be defined by them.

Today, see the beauty of you—all of you.

Daily Nutritional Information

Time	Amt.	Cal.	Fat gms	Protein gms	Carbs gms	Fiber gms
MORNING						
AFTERNOON						
EVENING						
TOTALS						

MY DAILY ACTIVITY

_____

_____

_____

_____

_____

_____

_____

_____

_____

> *"Aging always made me feel more substantial, as if I had more to offer other people and was more open."*
>
> —ᴇ ELLEN BARKIN

*a*s long as we keep breathing, we're going to get older. Rather then view this with horror, we can recognize a great opportunity. Along with gray hair and wrinkles, our years bring gifts of emotional and spiritual maturity.

What valuable lessons have we learned through the years? What experiences can we pass on to younger generations? If we embrace, rather than fight, the years, we can enrich not only our own lives, but also the lives of those around us.

Today, acknowledge the gifts that come with getting older.

Daily Nutritional Information

Time	Amt.	Cal.	Fat gms	Protein gms	Carbs gms	Fiber gms
MORNING						
AFTERNOON						
EVENING						
TOTALS						

MY DAILY ACTIVITY

_____

_____

_____

_____

_____

_____

_____

_____

_____

"Young man, I didn't fail 10,000 times trying to invent the light bulb, I simply found 10,000 ways that it wouldn't work!"

—THOMAS EDISON

*I*magine how different our world would look if Edison had quit after try number 8,764. His determination and focus are exactly what we need to fuel our own quest for wellness.

We may need to try different paths before we find one that works for us. The experimentation itself will serve us well—as we learn what doesn't work, we'll also see more clearly what does. All of our dedication and resolve will pay off when one day we flip the switch and . . . the light comes on.

Today, don't stop until you succeed.

Daily Nutritional Information

Time	Amt.	Cal.	Fat gms	Protein gms	Carbs gms	Fiber gms
MORNING						
AFTERNOON						
EVENING						
TOTALS						

MY DAILY ACTIVITY

_____

_____

_____

_____

_____

_____

_____

_____

_____

"Self-expression must pass into communication for its fulfillment."

— PEARL S. BUCK

"Oh, come on, you can have just one." "How long are you going to be on that diet?" "Can't you just have a taste?" Sometimes the biggest threat to our establishing a healthier lifestyle can be the good intentions of our loved ones. It's up to us to communicate what we need clearly and kindly to them.

We may have to say no repeatedly when people offer us inappropriate food, or ask them politely to stop offering. We may have to let people know in advance that we are avoiding certain foods. Every time we let the people around us know we are not budging from our commitment to health, we become stronger, healthier, and more focused.

Today, make sure you clearly communicate your needs.

Daily Nutritional Information

Time	Amt.	Cal.	Fat gms	Protein gms	Carbs gms	Fiber gms
MORNING						
AFTERNOON						
EVENING						
TOTALS						

MY DAILY ACTIVITY

> *"Dare to reach out your hand into the darkness, to pull another hand into the light."*
>
> —<small>∽ NORMAN B. RICE</small>

*a*s our bodies become stronger and leaner, as our minds blossom and fill with positive thoughts and self-esteem, we grow uniquely equipped to assist those just starting on the path to a healthier life.

The healthier we become, the more we have to give. We can offer viable solutions based on our experience, strength, and hope. We can model what healthy eating and living look like. We can encourage with quick praise and a well-timed kind word. We can give the kind of support that comes from someone who has been there, done that—and has a solution.

Today, share your experience with another.

Daily Nutritional Information

Time	Amt.	Cal.	Fat gms	Protein gms	Carbs gms	Fiber gms
MORNING						
AFTERNOON						
EVENING						
TOTALS						

MY DAILY ACTIVITY

> "It's the repetition of affirmations that leads to belief. And once that belief becomes a deep conviction, things begin to happen."
>
> —Ⴑ CLAUDE M. BRISTOL

*N*egative or positive, the words we say to ourselves day after day, year after year, become our beliefs. Recognizing this empowers us: If we create our beliefs, we can change them. Positive affirmations—short, present-tense statements that focus on what we want, not on what we don't— can help change our belief system. When we repeat these statements to ourselves, we reprogram our subconscious mind.

For example, affirming "Every day my body is becoming healthy and strong" can help facilitate physical healing; or, "Every day I am moving toward my ideal body weight" can foster patience with our weight loss. Whatever our situation, we can evoke positive change using the power of positive affirmations.

Today, create affirmations that will help you realize your goals.

Daily Nutritional Information

Time	Amt.	Cal.	Fat gms	Protein gms	Carbs gms	Fiber gms
MORNING						
AFTERNOON						
EVENING						
TOTALS						

MY DAILY ACTIVITY

_____

_____

_____

_____

_____

_____

_____

_____

_____

"Remember, [people] need laughter sometimes more than food."

—❧ ANNA FELLOWS JOHNSTON

We already know that laughter can help us heal if we are ill; let's not forget that it can help keep us feeling good, even when we're in the prime of health. People who feel good, physically and emotionally, tend to laugh more, but the reverse is also true.

If we can laugh—at the absurdities of life, at ourselves, or simply in pure joy—we can meet life's heaviest challenges more easily. When something throws us, we can pull out a favorite book or movie that we know will have us chuckling. Then we can get back to what we need to do with a balanced perspective and renewed energy.

Today, have a good laugh.

Daily Nutritional Information

Time	Amt.	Cal.	Fat gms	Protein gms	Carbs gms	Fiber gms
MORNING						
AFTERNOON						
EVENING						
TOTALS						

My Daily Activity

_____

_____

_____

_____

_____

_____

_____

_____

_____

"Keeping your body healthy is an expression of gratitude to the whole cosmos—the trees, the clouds, everything."

—THICH NHAT HANH

We're pretty good at finding all the flaws in our bodies. Too much fat here, not enough muscle there. Too short or too tall, too round or too thin. But our bodies carry us from place to place; they allow us to touch and smell and taste and see and hear. They let us be part of the great, wonderful world.

We owe it to our bodies to take care of them, with healthy food, regular exercise, and plenty of sleep. Doing that caretaking shows our appreciation for what we've been given: imperfect, yes, but wonderful bodies.

Today, do something good for your body.

Daily Nutritional Information

Time	Amt.	Cal.	Fat gms	Protein gms	Carbs gms	Fiber gms
MORNING						
AFTERNOON						
EVENING						
TOTALS						

My Daily Activity

> *"Every adversity carries within it the seed of equal or greater benefit."*
>
> —❧ NAPOLEON HILL

When faced with adversity, our first impulse may be to return to our old, unhealthy ways of coping, whether that's stuffing feelings with food, shutting out loved ones, or sinking into depression. We have to train ourselves to replace our self-destructive coping tools with healthy ones.

When adversity hits, we need to stick to our food plans more closely, connect with our support systems more frequently, and engage in our spiritual practices more regularly. Extra efforts keep our focus solid and make it easier for us to see past the discomfort of our present circumstances. When the adversity passes, we will emerge from it stronger, healthier, and wiser than before.

Today, view adversity as an opportunity for growth.

Daily Nutritional Information

Time	Amt.	Cal.	Fat gms	Protein gms	Carbs gms	Fiber gms
MORNING						
AFTERNOON						
EVENING						
TOTALS						

My Daily Activity

_____

_____

_____

_____

_____

_____

_____

_____

_____

_____

> *"Successful financial planning marries the meaning of life and the purpose of money."*
>
> —CHERIE D. PUTMAN

*M*oney is a tool that can enrich and empower us, as well as allow us to help others. Being financially healthy means planning in a way that supports our goals, respects our core values, and provides us with options.

Every wellness program should include a financial plan; it is one of the most loving gifts we can give to ourselves and our loved ones.

Today, have a financial plan.

Daily Nutritional Information

Time	Amt.	Cal.	Fat gms	Protein gms	Carbs gms	Fiber gms
MORNING						
AFTERNOON						
EVENING						
TOTALS						

MY DAILY ACTIVITY

_____

_____

_____

_____

_____

_____

_____

_____

"Every accomplishment starts with the decision to try."

—ANONYMOUS

Motivation can be a fair-weather friend—it's great when it's here, but when it leaves, it's gone. When our motivation disappears, how can we get it back? No matter how much we don't feel like it, we have to try.

Small, creative actions can get us going, such as posting sticky notes with reminders to drink enough water or printing out grocery lists. If we need a less subtle approach, perhaps we can invite a friend for a walk, making it more likely we'll take that walk ourselves. Once we get the momentum going, we'll find that our motivation is back and we're up and running.

Today, keep motivated.

Daily Nutritional Information

Time	Amt.	Cal.	Fat gms	Protein gms	Carbs gms	Fiber gms
MORNING						
AFTERNOON						
EVENING						
TOTALS						

MY DAILY ACTIVITY

> *"There are two mistakes one can make along the road to truth: not going all the way and not starting."*
>
> —⊙ BUDDHA

*I*t took effort to get started, to make a decision to live a healthier lifestyle. We knew that we were making a decision to change many habits and preferences in our lives, some of them small and some of them big. But we did it.

Now we have to keep making the decision to stay healthy, to keep the new habits and preferences we've acquired. We can't reach our goal of a healthier life and then just forget about it. It's a new life.

Today, no matter how far from (or close to) your wellness goals you are, recommit to them.

Daily Nutritional Information

Time	Amt.	Cal.	Fat gms	Protein gms	Carbs gms	Fiber gms
MORNING						
AFTERNOON						
EVENING						
TOTALS						

MY DAILY ACTIVITY

_____

_____

_____

_____

_____

_____

_____

_____

_____

> *"It takes courage to grow up and become who you really are."*
>
> —E. E. CUMMINGS

Our true selves are our best selves—happy, healthy, and serene. It takes courage to commit to being our best—eating healthy foods, exercising, and maintaining a good emotional balance. That sounds a little funny: Can it really be courageous to watch what we eat? As we proceed on this path to wellness, we can see that we have to be strong against a variety of forces that would undermine us.

Sometimes we sabotage ourselves with negative thoughts and weak moments. Sometimes those closest to us get in our way—with the best of intentions—by minimizing the problems we hope to correct, or by thinking they need to show their love with food. We can hold our heads up and be who we really are—no matter what the temptations.

Today, be your true self.

Daily Nutritional Information

Time	Amt.	Cal.	Fat gms	Protein gms	Carbs gms	Fiber gms
MORNING						
AFTERNOON						
EVENING						
TOTALS						

MY DAILY ACTIVITY

> "If you have no goal other than your personal happiness, you'll never achieve it. If you want to be happy, pursue something else vigorously and happiness will catch up with you."
>
> —ED DIENER

*H*appiness is like a lost cat that can't be found when we drive around looking for it, but then shows up when we give up and return home. Go figure.

Happiness is the byproduct of engaging in meaningful activities. Taking care of our health, counting our blessings, giving to others, finding fulfilling work—these are meaningful vehicles that carry happiness in their backseats. If we concentrate on enhancing our lives and the lives of others, one day we discover happiness has turned up at our front door all by itself.

Today, let happiness catch up with you.

Daily Nutritional Information

Time	Amt.	Cal.	Fat gms	Protein gms	Carbs gms	Fiber gms
MORNING						
AFTERNOON						
EVENING						
TOTALS						

MY DAILY ACTIVITY

> "Safeguard the health both of body and soul."
>
> —Ⓢ CLEOBULUS

*L*iving a balanced life brings multidimensional wellness, which means we need more than just good food and exercise to keep ourselves in top form—we also need to regularly tend to our overall well-being.

We can get so distracted by our loosening clothes or growing muscles that we forget about our emotional and spiritual health. At times, we need to gently remind ourselves that wellness also includes healthy things like close relationships and fulfilling activities. Tending to our inner health is just as important as tending to our outer health.

Today, take care of your whole self.

Daily Nutritional Information

Time	Amt.	Cal.	Fat gms	Protein gms	Carbs gms	Fiber gms
MORNING						
AFTERNOON						
EVENING						
TOTALS						

My Daily Activity

"Smoking cures weight problems . . . eventually."

—STEVEN WRIGHT

Sometimes our solutions end up being worse than our problems. How many of us, for example, lost weight by smoking cigarettes, taking diet pills, or starving ourselves? Ultimately, self-destructive "solutions" such as these end up becoming problems themselves. Even worse, they can eventually kill us.

Unlike false solutions, holistic wellness programs provide lasting, positive results. Whether we adopt a medically supervised food-and-exercise program, or join a support, twelve-step, or professional weight-loss group, we find real health and wellness when we treat the emotional, spiritual, and physical components of our total personhood with healthy actions.

Today, seek only real solutions.

Daily Nutritional Information

Time	Amt.	Cal.	Fat gms	Protein gms	Carbs gms	Fiber gms
MORNING						
AFTERNOON						
EVENING						
TOTALS						

MY DAILY ACTIVITY

_____

_____

_____

_____

_____

_____

_____

_____

_____

"I still need more healthy rest in order to work at my best. My health is the main capital I have and I want to administer it intelligently."

— ERNEST HEMINGWAY

Some of us find it difficult to relax when we look at our busy lives. We get overwhelmed when we see how much we need to do and what limited time we have to do it in. Personal interests, friendships, and catching up on sleep often run second to our "To Do" list.

The solution is to add "downtime" to our schedules. Treating downtime as a nonnegotiable task—just like going to work—allows us to become recharged mentally, physically, and spiritually. Ironically, adding downtime makes us even more productive in the long run because it gives us renewed clarity, energy, and enthusiasm.

Today, add downtime to your schedule.

Daily Nutritional Information

Time	Amt.	Cal.	Fat gms	Protein gms	Carbs gms	Fiber gms
MORNING						
AFTERNOON						
EVENING						
TOTALS						

MY DAILY ACTIVITY

_____

_____

_____

_____

_____

_____

_____

_____

_____

_____

"Every now and again, take a good look at something not made with hands—a mountain, a star, the turn of a stream. There will come to you wisdom and patience and solace and, above all, the assurance that you are not alone in the world."

—SIDNEY LOVETT

Spirituality is for everyone, whether we are atheist, agnostic, or deeply religious. Spirituality simply entails attaining a sense of connectedness with ourselves, with each other, and with a power greater than ourselves—whatever that means for each of us.

There is no right or wrong way to develop our spirituality. Some of us find peace through prayer, others through nature or other people. The only thing that matters is that we seek.

Today, seek inner peace.

Daily Nutritional Information

Time	Amt.	Cal.	Fat gms	Protein gms	Carbs gms	Fiber gms
MORNING						
AFTERNOON						
EVENING						
TOTALS						

MY DAILY ACTIVITY

_____

_____

_____

_____

_____

_____

_____

_____

_____

"As each day comes to us refreshed and anew, so does my gratitude renew itself daily. The breaking of the sun over the horizon is my grateful heart dawning upon a blessed world."

—ADABELLA RADICI

Spiritual practices are as individual as we are. Some of us find comfort, peace, and guidance in a formal place of worship; others find them in nature or on a yoga mat. No matter how, what, or whether we worship, there's one spiritual principle everyone can practice: gratitude.

From keeping a gratitude journal, to making lists of things we appreciate, to counting our blessings before bed, we can increase our joy by making gratitude part of our daily lives. Focusing on what we do have, rather than on what we don't, releases negative energy, connects us to our spirituality, and transforms our lives.

Today, have an attitude of gratitude.

Daily Nutritional Information

Time	Amt.	Cal.	Fat gms	Protein gms	Carbs gms	Fiber gms
MORNING						
AFTERNOON						
EVENING						
TOTALS						

MY DAILY ACTIVITY

> "A mind is like a parachute. It doesn't work if it is not open."
>
> —✑ FRANK ZAPPA

Many of us decided what we like and don't like in childhood and have never taken the time to examine those decisions. Early opinions can lead us automatically to dismiss potentially enjoyable experiences because we've already closed our minds. It's up to us to open our minds and become open for new experiences with familiar activities.

Maybe we've always said we hate certain vegetables, but when was the last time we actually tried them? Let's try them again, or try them prepared in a new way. If we tried meditation and found it boring, maybe we can give it another shot, adding some music or a change of scenery. We may have grown up, but we should never stop growing.

Today, have a new experience.

Daily Nutritional Information

Time	Amt.	Cal.	Fat gms	Protein gms	Carbs gms	Fiber gms
MORNING						
AFTERNOON						
EVENING						
TOTALS						

MY DAILY ACTIVITY

"Reality check: you can never, ever, use weight loss to solve problems that are not related to your weight."

—⟡ PHILLIP C. MCGRAW

W ho among us hasn't believed that one single event— whether that's losing weight, getting married, or getting a new job—would magically transform the rest of our lives? No one thing can deliver across-the-board happiness. We only find happiness when we live well on all levels: emotional, spiritual, and physical.

Our fitness goals are important to our living a healthier, better life, but achieving them won't make everything else in our life suddenly be perfect. If we're struggling with a job we don't like, or we have difficult relationships to deal with, they will still need our attention. Being healthier will help give us strength to deal with the other parts of our lives, but it won't erase our problems.

Today, live well on all levels.

Daily Nutritional Information

Time	Amt.	Cal.	Fat gms	Protein gms	Carbs gms	Fiber gms
MORNING						
AFTERNOON						
EVENING						
TOTALS						

MY DAILY ACTIVITY

> *"You've achieved success in your field when you don't know whether what you're doing is work or play."*
>
> —⟡ WARREN BEATTY

a healthy life doesn't stop with eating right and exercising; it includes finding work that is rewarding, stimulating, and enjoyable. When our work engages us, the line between work and play blurs, and we receive personal fulfillment along with our paycheck.

If our work doesn't engage us, we have choices. Whether we change jobs or simply our attitudes, every day has new opportunities to create satisfying work lives. We increase our happiness when we focus on maximizing our effectiveness, boosting our creativity, and setting and achieving personal goals in our professions.

Today, strive to blur the line between work and play.

Daily Nutritional Information

Time	Amt.	Cal.	Fat gms	Protein gms	Carbs gms	Fiber gms
MORNING						
AFTERNOON						
EVENING						
TOTALS						

My Daily Activity

> *"If you understand the force of intelligence in the body, its mechanical operation and structure, you can work on any part of the body you can reach with your hands."*
>
> —LAUREN BERRY

Our bodies pay the price of stress. Massage not only eases aches and pains, it also soothes our minds. Luckily, we don't have to go to a spa to get the benefits of a massage; we can take matters into our own hands—literally.

With a little research, we can learn to massage our own bodies safely to relieve the physical symptoms of stress, ease tension, and bring peace of mind. We can add to our massage with soothing scents, soft music, or a warm bath.

Today, try giving yourself some massage therapy.

Daily Nutritional Information

Time	Amt.	Cal.	Fat gms	Protein gms	Carbs gms	Fiber gms
MORNING						
AFTERNOON						
EVENING						
TOTALS						

My Daily Activity

_____

_____

_____

_____

_____

_____

_____

_____

_____

"My own prescription for health is less paperwork and more running barefoot through the grass."

—⟨ LESLIE GRIMUTTER

The papers keep piling up, no matter where we are. Bills to be paid, letters to answer, lists of what we need to do today, next week, this year. For many of us, the papers at home are nothing compared to what sits in our "in" basket at the office. We do our best to read and sign and dot all the "i's" we need to.

Unfortunately, we often find our free time consumed by that same paperwork. We'd not only be happier, we'd probably be more effective if we were to set aside the paperwork for at least a few hours and do something completely different—and enjoyable. We can run through the grass, or dance to our favorite music, or simply stretch toward the sun.

Today, put the paperwork aside for a while.

Daily Nutritional Information

Time	Amt.	Cal.	Fat gms	Protein gms	Carbs gms	Fiber gms
MORNING						
AFTERNOON						
EVENING						
TOTALS						

MY DAILY ACTIVITY

"Throughout my life, I've seen the difference that volunteering efforts can make in people's lives. I know the personal value of service as a local volunteer."

—JIMMY CARTER

When we give of our time, energy, and resources, we get a new perspective and gain a sense of purpose.

Volunteer work shows us that we are needed—and can make a difference for many others. How we volunteer is up to us. Some of us choose to volunteer in our area of expertise; others use volunteering as an opportunity to learn new skills. When we give of ourselves, we can be assured that we're getting even more in return.

Today, volunteer for something.

Daily Nutritional Information

Time	Amt.	Cal.	Fat gms	Protein gms	Carbs gms	Fiber gms
MORNING						
AFTERNOON						
EVENING						
TOTALS						

My Daily Activity

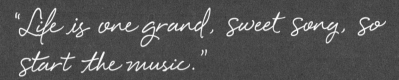

"Life is one grand, sweet song, so start the music."

—⏦ RONALD REAGAN

We all know that music provides the sound track to our lives, but we may not realize how profoundly it can positively affect our health.

Fast music awakens our minds; slow music helps them to sleep. Upbeat music moves our bodies; soft music soothes our stress. We can add music as an integral part of our spiritual practices to bring heightened awareness, connection, and serenity.

Today, tap into the power of music.

Daily Nutritional Information

Time	Amt.	Cal.	Fat gms	Protein gms	Carbs gms	Fiber gms
MORNING						
AFTERNOON						
EVENING						
TOTALS						

My Daily Activity

_____

_____

_____

_____

_____

_____

_____

_____

_____

> *"We visit others as a matter of social obligation. How long has it been since we have visited with ourselves?"*
>
> — MORRIS ADLER

*a*n important part of wellness is to carve out time to spend with that special someone—yourself. When we don't have enough Me Time, we risk becoming drained, irritable, and overwhelmed.

We may have to put Me Time on our calendars if our schedules don't naturally allow for it. It doesn't matter what we do, or how long we do it for, as long as it provides us space from others and recharges our batteries. We might take ourselves to the movies, shopping, or out to dinner. Or maybe we'll do nothing at all. Whatever we decide is good; we're on our own time.

Today, make a date with yourself.

Daily Nutritional Information

Time	Amt.	Cal.	Fat gms	Protein gms	Carbs gms	Fiber gms
MORNING						
AFTERNOON						
EVENING						
TOTALS						

MY DAILY ACTIVITY

_____

_____

_____

_____

_____

_____

_____

_____

_____

"Chase down your passion like it's the last bus of the night."

—ᴈ GLADE BYRON ADDAMS

The healthier we are in body and mind, the better the opportunity for being our best selves—and the greater our passion for living. When we feel good in body, mind, and spirit, we tap into the ability to meet life's challenges with grace and stamina.

How do we discover our passions? We only need to discover what we naturally love doing. What puts the wind in our sails? What energizes us? Once we recognize what our passions are, we can chase them with enthusiasm.

Today, live life with passion.

Daily Nutritional Information

Time	Amt.	Cal.	Fat gms	Protein gms	Carbs gms	Fiber gms
MORNING						
AFTERNOON						
EVENING						
TOTALS						

❤ MY DAILY ACTIVITY

_____

_____

_____

_____

_____

_____

_____

_____

_____

"A lot of people have gone further than they thought they could because someone else thought they could."

There is at least one person in everyone's life who has made a significant, positive impact. It can be a parent, a friend, a spouse, or a teacher. We may have known them all our lives or for only a short time. They make our lives better just by being in them, and leave us better people for having known them. Even if they are no longer living, their influence remains alive in us.

It's important to acknowledge those who helped make us the people we are today, who helped us through rough times, and whom we can always count on to be there when we need them.

Today, thank the special people in your life.

Daily Nutritional Information

Time	Amt.	Cal.	Fat gms	Protein gms	Carbs gms	Fiber gms
MORNING						
AFTERNOON						
EVENING						
TOTALS						

MY DAILY ACTIVITY

"One way to keep momentum going is to have constantly greater goals."

—ᴳ MICHAEL KORDA

When we've hit a goal, it's time to celebrate—and to set a new goal. There is no better time to refocus and find new motivation than when we're already racking up the successes. There are always greater dreams to dream, new challenges to tackle to keep moving forward. We haven't ended one path—we've just started another.

A healthy life is not an end point; it's a beginning of something wonderful.

Today, commit to keep moving forward.

Daily Nutritional Information

Time	Amt.	Cal.	Fat gms	Protein gms	Carbs gms	Fiber gms
MORNING						
AFTERNOON						
EVENING						
TOTALS						

MY DAILY ACTIVITY